ALLERGY EXPLOSION

ALLERGY EXPLOSION

Jo Revill

Kyle Cathie Limited

First published in Great Britain in 2007 by
Kyle Cathie Limited
122 Arlington Road, London NW1 7HP
general.enquiries@kyle-cathie.com
www.kylecathie.com

10 9 8 7 6 5 4 3 2 1

ISBN 978-1-85626-730-4

Text © 2007 Jo Revill
Book design © 2007 Kyle Cathie Limited

Editorial Director: Muna Reyal
Designer: Robert Updegraff
Copy editor: Hilary Boddie
Illustrations: Robert Updegraff
Production: Sha Huxtable and Alice Holloway

Jo Revill is hereby identified as the author of this work in accordance
with Section 77 of the Copyright, Designs and Patents Act 1988.

A Cataloguing In Publication record for this title is available
from the British Library.

Jacket reproduction by Oxted Colour Printers
Printed and bound in England by Martins the Printer

CONTENTS

Dedication

To my mother for her love and understanding,
and for her uncanny knack of always asking
exactly the right question, whatever the subject.

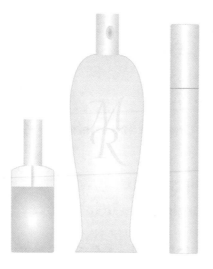

Acknowledgements

There are so many people who have helped me in the writing of this book: friends, family and many professionals who have given me time and their patience. Asthma UK is a charity that has been particularly helpful, and I'd like to thank the Guy's and St Thomas' NHS Trust for their help.

My agent Rob Shreeve has provided very clear advice, as ever, over what might interest the reader. The detailed work done by Muna Reyal at Kyle Cathie and her comments in guiding me through some of the more abstruse points have been instructive and enlightening; her enthusiasm kept us both going over some long weekends! I would like to voice my appreciation for my employer, The Observer, which gave me the time to write this. They did so, as ever, with understanding and supportiveness, and I owe thanks to two particular colleagues, Jan Thompson and Kamal Ahmed.

My family has endured months of endless discussions about allergies, and I think my children Flora and Seb now know far too much about hayfever and dermatitis. As for my husband Michael, his endless patience in having books and papers scattered around the house should earn him a special medal. He has no allergy that I have yet been able to diagnose.

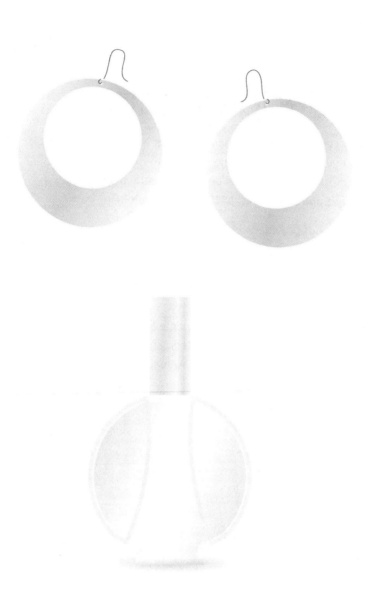

INTRODUCTION

Citrus fruit, cat spit, alder pollen, milk, latex, formaldehyde, fresh paint, nickel-plated earrings. The list of substances that can trigger a host of unpleasant and painful symptoms grows longer every year. Just as mankind is emerging from the shadow of typhoid, polio and other deadly infectious diseases that plagued us at the beginning of the last century, we are becoming ever more burdened with a new kind of disease – allergy. Thankfully, most of these conditions are not fatal but they can have a profound impact on your life, or the life of your child. They are, for the most part, life-long, chronic illnesses for which there is no quick-fix cure. One in three people in the UK now develops some form of allergy, and the rate is increasing.

I wrote this book because I wanted to understand why the rates of allergies were soaring around the world. As a health journalist, it seemed to me that the story of allergies had been untold and that more needed to be understood about the sharp rise in cases. I hope this book can go some way to explaining what we currently know about the different conditions, how they are related to each other, and to the best of our knowledge, which treatments actually work.

Britain, America, New Zealand and Australia have the highest allergy rates in the world – some five times greater than those seen in the former Soviet states of Georgia and Uzbekistan. But then there are some strange anomalies – some of the Aboriginal tribes are also beginning to experience extremely high rates of asthma. In Chapter Two, I try to set out what is known so far about the reasons behind the increase in the prevalence of eczema, hayfever and asthma, but also in more unusual conditions such as peanut allergy. The book explores the 'hygiene hypothesis' – the concept that our obsession with cleanliness and killing germs has left us, and our children, with immune systems which cannot now differentiate between a real threat such as a virus and a fake threat, such as a grain of pollen or a strand of cat hair. Increasingly, it looks as if our individual predisposition to allergies is programmed in us, within the first year of life. There is a genetic influence certainly, but the foods you eat as a baby may be the key to your immune system developing some robust defences against pollen, house-dust mites and other allergens.

When it comes to scientific research, these are exciting times, thanks to our genetic knowledge and new lab techniques. These days, researchers are also able to tell us far more about what is happening in human cells when they become sensitised to an allergen. Today, many more people are allergy sufferers but we are still at the beginning of the journey of discovery into the cause and pattern of these allergies and it will be a good few years before we really understand the complex interaction between our environment, our genes, our food and our health. I have spoken to many different experts about their attempts to unravel these uncertainties, and this book is aimed at explaining some of those complexities in language that I hope is clear but not patronising.

It is increasingly clear that the changing climate is also going to contribute to a bigger burden of illness across the world. In Europe, doctors are beginning to see patients who have never previously suffered from hayfever exhibiting symptoms. This is because new plants are able to grow in a warmer climate and because the pollen load is also changing. Not only are the key proteins within the pollen becoming stronger, but they are also appearing earlier in the year and disappearing at a later stage. The same goes for insects, with Germany having seen a record number of insect stings in 2004 after a summer of record heat.

The combination of environmental and health factors makes it imperative for governments to act now, before the burden of illness becomes any greater. The good news is that the World Health Organisation is charting the rise in allergies and has helped to raise the profile of such illnesses which lead to an enormous amount of disability. In the UK, we spend £900m on asthma treatment but a staggering £1.2bn on incapacity benefit for asthma patients, since the condition makes it impossible for many sufferers to work. There are no cures for these chronic conditions. You can hope and pray that your child grows out of eczema or that the bad cough your teenager has every night is not the tell-tale sign of asthma, but there's precious little you can actually do about it, in terms of a cure.

INTRODUCTION

The scale of neglect that sufferers face is huge. It is almost unbelievable that every week in Britain, more than 800,000 children wake up at night wheezing because of their asthma. That means that more than 800,000 adults also wake up, their lives disrupted by a condition that should be entirely manageable for the vast majority of families. As for the children themselves, the fear of an asthma attack, of being unable to breathe, is one which can dominate their thoughts, cause depression and harm their education. But because of a lack of funding and a lack of specialist support, many families struggle for years trying to help their children, not knowing how to control the symptoms or prevent them from becoming isolated from other children. In the USA, many poor families simply cannot afford to buy the medications they need to control their condition and consequently the death rate remains far too high. Asthma is the epidemic of our times.

Into this void comes an entire army of complementary health practitioners to offer diagnoses and treatments of very doubtful nature. Some private allergy clinics do carry out the right kinds of tests and essentially offer what should be offered by the National Health Service. But there are a whole range of others – naturopaths, kinesiologists and homeopaths – where there is no firm evidence to show that their expensive methods work. People going to these clinics sometimes are given wrong diagnoses which will mean that it takes that much longer to get the right answers. One of the central messages of this book is that people with allergies must be aware of the dangers of unconventional treatment. The first port of call should always be the family doctor, who will know about the process of diagnosis and should offer a referral to hospital specialists if necessary.

One of the hardest areas to investigate is food allergies. No one really knows how prevalent they are, or whether or not the rate is increasing, although this does seem to be the case for peanut and milk allergies. The problem is the symptoms can differ enormously from individual to individual and the only real way to uncover an allergy or intolerance is to go on an elimination diet which takes several weeks to follow rigorously. The difference it can make to your life, however, is huge – many people say that the feelings of lethargy, cramps and bloatedness disappear once they find the source of their problem.

Children need special help and this is important when it comes to hayfever, eczema, peanut allergy and asthma. The many websites offering reliable information can assist parents in finding out far more about conditions and children themselves can learn how to cope in an emergency, such as anaphylactic shock. It's not nice to think that a child with a peanut allergy might have to use a shot of adrenaline injected into the leg, but it's absolutely essential until doctors can find another way of dealing with it.

There are, however, some rays of hope on the horizon. There is, for example, a new vaccine which now works for people who find every other hayfever medication fairly ineffective. For patients with asthma, the medication has improved a great deal, so that the underlying inflammation of the lungs can be tackled, rather than simply waiting for the breathlessness to begin. There is also a concerted attempt to make patients 'experts' in their own condition, so that they can work with doctors and nurses to improve not only their own care, but that of other patients too.

In the chapters on individual allergies, I've tried to explain how to get an accurate diagnosis and then give an explanation of the different treatments. Access to the therapies will depend on where you live and, in some cases, whether you are able to go privately for them. But for many allergy sufferers there are some more simple solutions, which include trying to avoid the allergen in the first place. If you are a hayfever sufferer, for example, understanding how pollen spreads over the day and how to prevent it coming into the house will be crucial to you mastering the condition.

People are searching for cures, searching for answers. This book attempts to answer some of the questions about the reasons for the increase and what you can do about individual allergies. Above all, the need for good dialogue with your doctor is paramount. When it comes to tackling any of these conditions, ignorance is indeed your worst enemy. Find out as much as you can about your, or your child's, condition and you are halfway there to beating it.

13

PART ONE
ABOUT ALLERGIES

CHAPTER ONE
HOW ALLERGIES WORK

How is it possible that we can react in such different ways to chemicals and substances that we come into contact with every day and which have been around for centuries? What seems so puzzling is that even close members of the same family can experience wildly differing reactions to identical substances. And why are we now so sensitive to particles such as pollen, given that our immune systems have evolved over thousands of years to deal with any kind of foreign bodies that we might breathe in?

In the last twenty years, there has been a significant amount of scientific progress made in relation to our understanding of what happens within cells when you have an allergic response. The more that is understood about the chain of events that is triggered by a piece of pollen or a house-dust mite, the more we can begin to unravel the tangled relationship between the genetic and the environmental factors that are involved.

The term allergy derives from the Greek words *allos*, meaning other, and *ergon* meaning work. The term itself is quite broad and can cover any kind of reaction involving the immune system, however, for most sufferers, it involves a sensitivity to a particular chemical or substance. This is known as a Type 1 hypersensitivity.

It is the job of our immune system to protect us from foreign invaders, known as antigens. From the moment a baby emerges from the womb, he or she is exposed to all kinds of bacteria and viruses that would prove fatal were the body not equipped with an awesomely sophisticated way of repelling them. The cold viruses that swirl around and infect us every winter, for example, are mostly harmless because the body can recognise the invader and mount a defence.

When a germ is breathed in, or enters the bloodstream, our immune system produces antibodies – molecules designed to latch on to particular viruses or bacteria and disable them before they can do harm. This is fine when the body needs to protect itself from an antigen such as a pneumococcal bacteria. However, in the case of allergies, antibodies are marshalled against the wrong enemy. They go into battle against substances that are very common and which may be all around us, such as grass pollen.

IgE, the villain

Every allergic response begins with sensitisation – the period when the cells first produce a particular antibody response to what they think is an invader. The chief villain of the piece is an antibody known as immunoglobulin E, or IgE. This protein molecule, discovered in 1911, is common in most allergic reactions and its levels can be measured through a blood test. Immunoglobulin evolved in humans as a way of fighting off parasites, such as ringworm, and levels of it are still high in those living in tropical countries where there are parasitic illnesses.

A chemical or substance that produces an allergic response is known as an allergen. As we will see, this could be the coating on a piece of pollen, mould from a fir tree, or the saliva of a cat. An allergen is not a particular substance in itself, but really a description of the way people react to it. A feather-filled pillow can mean luxurious sleep to some of us; for others, it equates to a night of misery, wheezing and a constantly runny nose.

Normally, when a foreign body such as a piece of pollen is inhaled, the body's reaction is for certain cells to absorb the molecule and then, as part of the normal immune response, to expose it to other cells. This would include 'showing' it to the important white blood cells known as T-lymphocytes, which act as the infantry of the immune fighting system. Through a series of changes, these cells are then transformed into plasma cells that secrete, or send out antibodies.

During a normal immune reaction, our plasma cells produce antibodies known as immunoglobulin M – a chemical that fights off antigens such as the cold virus. However, in an allergic individual, something goes awry. The allergen is mistaken for a hostile piece of protein, and triggers a response involving immunoglobulin E (IgE). A combination of faulty genes and environmental factors means that the body is 'over-responding' to allergens. It is a case of mistaken identity that can have long-term consequences for the sufferer.

When IgE is released, it binds itself to the receptors of certain cells – rather in the way a ship docks in a port. There are two types of cells involved: mast cells, which are produced by the bone marrow and are scattered throughout the body, and basophils, a type of white blood cell found in the blood. Once the cells' receptors have been taken over by IgE, they are effectively coated with the antibody.

After the first reaction

The first stage of an allergic response is known as sensitisation – the first time when IgE is produced in response to a common and usually harmless substance.

However, after this has happened once, the body is in some way then primed to over-react the next time that it is exposed to the same allergen. The IgE-coated cells are re-activated. It is as if the cell has a kind of memory and subsequently produces a more rapid and aggressive response to what it perceives to be a great threat.

There are several stages in a reaction, but the most important one is known as degranulation. This is where the mast cells start to break up and release some of their granules, which contain chemicals known as inflammatory mediators which end up in surrounding tissues. It is this process that appears to cause so many of the problems associated with an allergic response. A cascade effect is produced, with chemical after chemical being released as part of the defence system. One of those released is histamine, which plays such an important role in hayfever. The mast cells also release what is known as messenger chemicals and, in particular, some which are called leukotrienes. These are damaging, and go on to cause further inflammation in different tissues.

This whole chain of chemical events results in several unwanted effects such as the widening of blood vessels in the nose, the stimulation of nerves, bronchoconstriction in the lungs (where the airways start to narrow) and contraction of smooth muscle in the gut. The symptoms that are experienced in allergies – the runny nose, itchiness, stomach problems or the breathlessness – all come from this complex immune reaction.

Early and late phase response

The acute phase of the reaction usually happens within fifteen minutes of exposure to an allergen, but you can also then get what doctors call a ' late phase response'. The different white blood cells can travel to the area affected by the allergen, for example, the nose, lungs or throat or perhaps the respiratory tract, sometimes four to six hours after the allergen has first affected the area. This initial reaction may only last for one to two days or it can go on for days or even weeks. This response is different from those described in the previous paragraph. The body is going through a sustained allergic response which causes more reaction in the bronchial tubes of the lungs, a build up of fluid in the tissues and yet more inflammation.

What IgE does is 'teach' the immune system to respond to allergens by triggering the release of these chemicals which cause both early and delayed reactions.

Do allergies run in families?

Since the 1920s, doctors have known that asthma is passed down in families, suggesting at least some kind of genetic basis to the disease. But in those days, they also imagined that there were strong psychological causes: patients were labelled as 'asthmatic types' and often their parents were told they had created the breathing difficulties by making them anxious and stressed. We now know this not to be the case, although stress does exacerbate the condition.

Just because parents have allergies, it doesn't mean that their children will go on to inherit the same conditions or even suffer to the same extent. Identical twins, who share the same genes, both carry the same propensity to be allergic but may have different reactions to the same substances.

Atopy, from the Greek word meaning placelessness, is the term doctors use to describe an underlying predisposition to have an allergy. A person who is atopic is someone who is much more likely to develop allergies. It does run in families and it seems that for each close family member who already suffers from an allergy, your own chances of having one is increased twofold. In Chapter Three, I'll describe what parents can do to try and protect their children from developing allergies.

Atopy or atopic syndrome, as it is sometimes called, is usually diagnosed by seeing higher than normal levels of IgE in the blood and this can be demonstrated by a skin-prick test which will show sensitivity to common allergens. Doctors often rely on talking to the parents of a child about their family history to ascertain whether there is likely to be atopy. It has been found to be more common in red-haired people for reasons that are not fully understood.

In the past decade, great strides have been made in understanding the root causes of allergy thanks to new laboratory techniques that open up the world of individual cells and their components. Through the latest DNA technology, we can now see how different cells interact with each other and, in the case of allergies, how they provoke the inflammation that causes so many varying symptoms.

Allergy is a very complex phenomenon involving many different factors and some scientists believe it will be several decades before the underlying causes are fully understood. With heart disease, the new scanning techniques allow cardiologists to make fairly accurate diagnoses in a way which wasn't possible twenty years ago, but that is not at all the case for allergy specialists. Symptoms vary from person to person, which has the added complication of making it much harder to carry out big clinical studies where researchers can compare the cases of thousands of patients to see which genes may be involved. The other complication is that even if you carry the allergy genes, they may need an environmental trigger – such as pollution or cigarette smoke – to be activated and you would then need to know if the trigger had to happen at a particular point in your life, such as in your early or teenage years.

We know that if one parent has an allergy, then the child has a 40 per cent chance of developing one too. If both parents are allergic to something, then that risk rises to 70–80 per cent. However, the child's allergy may be completely different to those of their parents. This inheritance factor has been very much noted in asthma studies, where a mother with the condition is more likely than the father to pass it on to the child.

It is likely that within the next decade there will be far more genetic information which will enable us to map out the relationship between a particular 'allergy' gene, environmental factors such as cigarette smoking and the role of diet, but at the moment that is impossible. Pharmaceutical companies talk about a 'genomics revolution' in which new medications will be created that target particular genetic flaws, but in 2007 that remains just a distant hope.

 At the scientific coalface

At his laboratory in Houston, Texas, USA, Roberto Adachi is looking at the inner working of the mast cell. He believes it is the key to the understanding of allergies.

Mast cells are interesting because they are hugely important in the body's armoury as they fight off bacterial infections, but they are also a key part of the allergic response. Adachi, a critical care medicine doctor at the Houston Veterans Affairs Medical Center, explains: 'We are looking for a way to retain the cell's ability to fight infection while shutting down the parts responsible for allergy and inflammation. It is a process of first understanding each individual part, then learning how the parts work together and finally determining how you can change the way they work.'

Mast cells are found right through the airways, the lining of the nose and the stomach. But when they begin to degranulate, chemicals are released which cause the inflammation of tissues, and thus the symptoms. Adachi's team is exploring the degranulation process in the hope of finding a means of shutting it down. He is particularly interested in the final phase of degranulation, when the granule membrane fuses with the cell membrane and releases its contents. So far, Adachi's laboratory has detected nine protein components of the machinery involved in the final step.

'We have isolated each component and studied it and now we want to know how they work together' he says. 'Our final goal is to have a mast cell that will still defend us against bacterial infection but will be unable to hurt us.'

The all-important T-cells

Much of the genetic research being carried out is looking at how our DNA is affected by T cells (the white blood cells that defend us from infection). In particular, there is a lot of focus on what are known as the T 'helper' cells. These provide assistance to other cells by recognising foreign bodies and also producing the different substances that set off an immune response. When a baby is born, these cells are like a blank canvas. They are in a 'naïve state' and have not yet fully formed into either TH1 or TH2 cells.

The TH1 cells are there to fight off infectious diseases and these are the ones that will respond to any dirt or bacteria or virus that a baby or young child comes into contact with. The TH2 cells play a triggering role in activating the cells that produce IgE.

There has been growing evidence to suggest that in people who are atopic, the TH2 cells predominate but no one is yet clear why. Some scientists believe it is due to the fact that if children are not sufficiently exposed to bacteria and dirt, the TH1 cells never develop properly. This means that the TH2 line becomes dominant, causing a sensitivity to allergic reactions which cannot be reversed. This theory that a lack of exposure to dirt or particular bacteria in the early years is key to developing an allergy will be fully explored in Chapter Two.

Age of onset

Many allergies begin in childhood, but the good news is that some 'classic allergies', such as atopic eczema, can disappear as the child gets older. It may be that as the immune system matures, there are changes in the cells' response to common substances which work in the sufferer's favour. Children can grow out of asthma, although experts say that it is a condition which is chronic, or long-term, and may reoccur at any stage in the future.
It is also true that some people do become asthmatic for the first time when they are adults.

Sometimes new allergies are seen in older people, simply because they are being exposed to specific allergens for the first time. One case reported in Italy in 2002, involved a group of around 2,000 citizens living north of Milan, who suddenly began to develop hayfever and asthma. It turned out that they had suddenly been exposed to two new airborne allergens, ragweed and birch pollen. Although the individuals probably carried some genetic sensitivity to these pollens, it had never been a problem until the new pollen grains wafted in to their area, due to environmental changes. Cases such as these are likely to become more widespread as global warming changes the pattern of the spread of pollen (see Chapter Four, Hayfever, page 59).

CHAPTER TWO
THE RISE IN ALLERGIES

Scattered along the archipelago of the Torres Strait in Australia lie 248 islands. With fifteen indigenous communities, this beautiful region is geographically isolated from the mainland as well as from other islands by vast stretches of water. It is the last place in the world you would associate with illness, given its warm climate, rich marine ecosystem and abundance of wildlife. But the islanders who live here are suffering from an epidemic of illness that doctors are struggling to understand. From a young age, their children start to wheeze and become out of breath if they over-exert themselves. The classic symptoms of asthma that we associate with modern life have become theirs too.

It has been suspected for a while that children of indigenous groups might be starting to suffer from allergies that their neighbouring white communities have had for some time, but no one was quite sure. Back in 2000, researchers from Queensland University visited the region and went from house to house, questioning the local residents about their health. They used the standard questionnaire that is now used by every health team in the world investigating childhood asthma. Interviews with the parents or carers were carried out mainly by local health workers who could clearly explain exactly what they were trying to achieve.

What they found from their survey astonished them. These children, most of them Melanesian, had a 20 per cent prevalence rate of asthma symptoms. This was higher than is seen in black American children (13.4 per cent) and slightly higher than other Australian children, whose rates range from 17–19.5 per cent.

Even more worryingly, many of the children who were wheezing said that it was bad enough to disturb their sleep and one-quarter of them said it actually affected their speech. The poorer the family, the more likely the child was to have had up to three asthma attacks in the last twelve months. One mainland community, Bamaga, had the highest proportions of all, while Umagico, just three kilometres away, had the lowest rate. No one can understand what is going on in these islands, where there is barely any air pollution and no genetic history of sensitivity.

What could have led to such an enormous increase in the number of children with allergies in such a short space of time? Many doctors describe it as an epidemic, due to the sheer numbers involved (even though, strictly speaking, epidemics are caused by infectious diseases and most allergies are life-long, incurable conditions).

Pinning down the causes of this rise is proving difficult. Some researchers have blamed modern, dust-free homes, while others have pointed to diet. But as yet, there is no real understanding why countries such as Australia, New Zealand, the USA and Britain have some of the highest rates of allergies in the world.

Asthma, one of the most serious and debilitating forms of allergy, is a prime example. It has increased by around 160 per cent globally in the last twenty years, with the rates of increase varying from between 3–20 per cent per annum around the world. In the UK, asthma is now the most common long-term condition in children, affecting one in ten. A staggering one in five households will have someone with the condition and one person will die from it every seven hours.

And it isn't just asthma which is giving cause for concern. Eczema, hayfever, food allergies, sensitivity to chemicals and animals, severe reactions to some metals – all of these allergies are steadily becoming more widespread. Hayfever, also called allergic rhinitis, has been diagnosed in an estimated 14 per cent of American adults, or nearly thirty million people. Since 1996, in America, the number of children affected by hayfever has risen from 6 per cent to 9 per cent, according to the National Center for Health Statistics. All allergies seem to be on the rise it seems, but according to Dr Marc Rothenberg, Director of Allergy and Immunology at Cincinnati Children's Hospital, 'it's not just that more kids have allergies. The severity of those allergies has also increased'.

Europe, where standards of living have risen fast in the past three decades, has seen a corresponding threefold increase in hayfever, asthma and eczema. One in three Europeans is now thought to have some kind of sensitivity to an allergen. Hayfever now affects one in five Europeans and the rate is growing as the pollen seasons change. Eczema, or atopic dermatitis as it is sometimes known, is seen in around 12 per cent of people across the continent and the costs of treating them are also soaring – the latest estimate is that an annual £22bn is spent both on medical care and in lost productivity, due to symptoms.

29

The World Health Organisation warned back in 2003 that the situation was becoming serious. 'Europe is facing an epidemic of allergic diseases and asthma, which have steadily increased in recent years,' said Dr Roberto Bertollini, one of the organisation's directors. 'In most countries in the European region, from the mid-1970s to the mid-1990s, the prevalence of asthma symptoms in children was reported to increase by 200 per cent, although in some parts of the region, such as Italy and the United Kingdom, the increase may have abated. In the European Union, allergic disease is the most common chronic illness of childhood, and in some areas it can be estimated to affect more than one child in four.'

Among the many factors associated with asthma and allergies, the environmental consequences of climate change have recently attracted the attention of scientists and the public health community. Changes in temperature and precipitation patterns may alter the length and timing of the growing season of plants producing pollen. On average, the length of the pollen season in Europe increased by ten to eleven days over the last thirty years. Longer and more intense exposure to pollen can raise both the number of allergic episodes and the demand for healthcare.

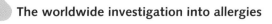 **The worldwide investigation into allergies**

Much of our knowledge about allergies comes from a huge study in children across the world, known as ISAAC, the International Study of Asthma and Allergies in Childhood. A unique project, begun in 1991, it has now looked at more than 720,000 children in fifty-six countries, using both simple, written questionnaires and more intensive studies to chart the rise in allergic conditions. It focuses on two age group, six to seven year olds and thirteen to fourteen year olds, to try and find out how such illnesses have developed.

The first phase showed the prevalence of asthma symptoms in children across the world, including populations that had never been studied before. Major differences in the rates are seen between countries, much of which is thought to be due to pollution levels. And it has also charted really alarming rises in the rates of allergies.

In Bangkok, for example, doctors found that over a six-year period there has been a fourfold increase in wheezing and a threefold increase in allergic rhinitis (hayfever) among children. The rates of eczema, however, stayed stable. In a 1998 paper on the subject, paediatricians warned: 'Results of this study indicate that allergic diseases are perhaps the most common childhood diseases in Thailand and could lead to a substantial economic loss for the country.'

Some countries have been able to find out a great deal about whether their children are receiving effective treatment for asthma. In Australia, one in four primary school children and one in seven teenagers currently suffer from the condition and it is the most common cause of hospital admissions for children between the ages of five and fourteen.

According to the ISAAC results, Australia has the world's third highest prevalence of a wheezing cough in thirteen to fourteen year olds. It has also showed doctors that there is a continuing lack of effective treatment of asthma. Among thirteen to fourteen year olds who had more than twelve episodes of wheeze per year, only 43 per cent were taking regular preventive medication.

The ISAAC studies have been carried out in three phases and the results from the Phase Three studies are coming through now. This latest phase was a hugely complex task, completed in 2002–2003, in which researchers carried out a cross-sectional questionnaire survey of 193,404 children, aged six to seven years from sixty-six centres in thirty-seven countries, and 304,679 children aged thirteen to fourteen years from 106 centres in fifty-six countries, chosen from a random sample of schools in a defined geographical area.

A paper published in August 2006 in the British medical journal, *The Lancet*, gave the latest data. It contained both bad and good news.

It showed that in most areas, younger children were experiencing more allergic symptoms than ever before. However, among the teenagers living in areas with high rates of asthma, such as Britain and Australia, researchers saw that there had actually been a decrease in asthma symptoms. It is not clear whether this is the result of teenagers receiving better medication and care, or whether it is due to environmental factors such as reduced air pollution.

The war on dirt

We live in a hygiene-obsessed society. Everywhere around us you can see the war on dirt: antibacterial soaps, disposable handwipes, special anti-germ lotions to rub on a knee as soon as the child has a cut. Keeping clean has become an international obsession, but could it possibly be responsible for the huge rise in allergic conditions?

Many doctors think so, and they call it the hygiene hypothesis (see page 32). The belief stems from the fact that as we become cleaner, we also appear to become more susceptible to allergens. It is possible that one of the consequences of our modern fear of dirt is the increase of life-long conditions.

As we discussed in the previous chapter, the immune system is key to the development of allergies. We know that when a baby is born, he or she has a full set of T cells which are waiting to develop so that they can fight off bacteria. Scientists believe that if infants and young children are not exposed to dirt at an early stage of their life, the T cells will develop more into TH2 cells, responsible for the production of the antibody IgE which triggers an allergic response. It may also be the case that some people are genetically predisposed to having more TH2 cells and that they only need to be exposed to a trigger, such as ragweed pollen, to be tipped over the edge into an allergy.

What seems to be important is that the T cells in a child are activated fully from birth so that they have the chance to develop into TH1 cells. These fight off invading bacteria and help to curtail the amount of TH2 cells. The question is, what substance or food do children need to be exposed to in order to allow this to happen?

The hygiene hypothesis

In developed countries such as Britain, the diseases that were once the major killers such as smallpox, typhoid fever and cholera have disappeared. It is rare for a child these days to die of an infectious disease. Thanks to clean water, antibiotics and vaccines, the terrible epidemics of the past have disappeared in prosperous countries. The same cannot be said for the poorer parts of the world, where gastrointestinal infections still kill many children before the age of five.

However, some people think that our success in shielding people from infection and from parasites is exactly what is now doing us harm. The imbalance in the T cells may be triggering a host of illnesses, including allergies. Others believe that it can also lead to an increase in autoimmune diseases such as rheumatoid arthritis. Is the attempt to wipe out infections, seen in communities as diverse as the Aborigines and the Hispanic Americas, causing this rise?

David Strachan, Professor in Public Health at St George's Hospital Medical School in London, is the man who first came up with the theory that we know now as the 'hygiene hypothesis'. In 1989, he put forward his ideas in a scientific paper which suggested that our preoccupation with cleanliness and hygiene might make it easier for allergies to become more widespread. Initially, this theory was received with huge scepticism. Since then, however, as researchers have struggled to disprove it, his explanation has gained quite a following. The discovery, in the early 1990s, of the way in which TH1 and TH2 cells work and the fact that you can build up a natural immunity with TH1 that somehow suppressed the TH2 responses gave his ideas increased credibility, as it laid down a proper scientific pathway in which it might work.

In that early paper, he stated that our insistence on being clean and free of germs was actually preventing members of a family from cross-infecting each other and that this was contributing to the rise in allergies. He wrote: 'Over the past century, declining family size, improved household amenities and higher standards of personal cleanliness have reduced opportunities for cross-infection in young families. This may have resulted in more widespread clinical expression of atopic disease.'

THE RISE IN ALLERGIES

Professor Strachan formulated his theory because, like others, he was attempting to explain the exponential rise in allergic conditions that he was witnessing firsthand through the patients he was seeing in his clinics. At the time, he felt that a number of factors affecting the home and the size of the family were leading to the rise in allergies. Ten years later, he was focusing more attention on the idea that some common infections, caught in childhood, might play a role in protecting us from developing allergies.

Currently, in 2007, he is focusing on the role that is played by the intestinal flora, the bacteria which reside in our guts and which play a vital part in fighting off infections and disease throughout our lives. This is an area that interests many scientists and the relationship between nutrition in early life and later allergies is being investigated worldwide (see Chapter Three, Preventing Allergies pages 43–55).

For Professor Strachan, the difficulty with the hygiene hypothesis is actually pinning down the specific explanations underlying the original observation. 'We think there may be something in the way all unhygienic conditions actually protect us from allergens and, since 1989, an enormous amount of research has been done into possible causes,' he says. 'I do think that allergies may be the price we pay for a better standard of living and a better general health.' And therein lies the dilemma – that the bacteria we may need to be exposed to in order to avoid allergies may also be dangerous to us, in other circumstances. 'The truth is that we could find that whatever we do to protect ourselves against allergies, could be harmful in some other ways.'

As he points out, research hasn't been able to show us any specific illnesses acquired from siblings or others that actually produce a protective effect. The big studies carried out to look at whether particular infections, such as measles, are protective have been inconclusive. He believes that whatever is happening to children to make them more prone to allergies may be happening after the first twelve to eighteen months of life.

For years it has been known that growing up on a farm can be protective and some work has been done into looking at children's proximity to animals. But like many areas of investigation into allergies, there is conflicting evidence about whether or not growing up around animals such as cats and dogs is a good idea. Many doctors advise that babies should not be allowed near cats for the first six months of life – even visiting a friend's house with a cat, they argue, could be putting the baby at risk of developing an allergy. However, in a large study which began in 1980, and still continues, doctors at the Henry Ford Health System in Detroit, USA, found that children who grew up with a pet in the first year of life were significantly less likely to develop allergies to that animal later in life. The same study also showed that these children were also less likely to react to some common allergens such as ragweed, grass and dust. The jury is still out on this.

Professor Strachan believes it may be decades before we fully understand allergies:

'I have been at this now for almost twenty years and what progress has been made? We really have not moved it forward much in that time, partly because it hasn't enjoyed massive amounts of investment in the research. Of course, there could be a breakthrough in understanding allergy but I think it is likely that I will retire in fifteen years and we will still not know what is going on.'

Germany – the East/West divide

The reunification of Germany on 3 October 1990 was one of the most significant changes in the political geography of Europe in the 20th century. As the Berlin Wall came tumbling down, the old days of the Cold War finally disappeared, and the East/West divide was replaced with different national interests. It had been known for some time that, quite apart from their political differences, East and West Germany had hugely contrasting societies, economies and healthcare systems. The reunification of these lands offered scientists something else – the chance to see what might be going on with allergies if lifestyles of a whole country started to change.

Back in 1990, Dr Ursula Kramer, an allergy specialist, decided to look at the rates of allergies across the divide. 'We knew there was a lot of air pollution in East Germany at that time,' she explained. 'Our main hypothesis was that we would see more allergies as a result.' But to her surprise, the opposite was the case. A comparison between thousands of children growing up in both countries showed that the more modern, western society of West Germany, where the air was far cleaner, had far higher rates of allergy. In fact, the conditions that the East Germans were living in appeared to be somehow protecting their children from developing these chronic conditions.

In the decade following reunification, the researchers then had a chance to do follow-up studies in the same regions looking at the same factors to see what might be going on. They looked at thousands of children at the age of six and found that, as the standard of living improved in the poorer regions of eastern Germany, so its rates of childhood eczema and asthma increased. This wasn't just down to better diagnosis – the same criteria for diagnosis were applied to both groups.

Many theories abounded as to what had caused lower rates of atopy in the East. Was it the fact that children tended to have more exposure to dirt at an early age? Was it that they had coal fires, rather than central heating? Some thought that it was linked to the fact that so many children were put into large nurseries at less than a year of age as their parents went to work in factories. This meant that they picked up dozens of different bugs, strengthening the immune system in the process.

The studies, involving 28,888 children in all, showed that the more educated the parents, the more likely the children were to have been diagnosed with an allergy and also to be showing the symptoms. In particular, they were more sensitised to grass pollen and to house-dust mites.

The studies raised many other questions because there were factors that were not looked at. The research had been designed specifically to look at the role of air pollution, so the diet of the children, for example, was not studied in depth.

In conclusion, Dr Kramer, who is a researcher at the Institut für Umweltmedizinische Forschung in Dusseldorf, Germany, said: 'We saw a number of things – that children put into daycare centres at an early stage had less allergies than those who were not. Those with older siblings also had fewer allergies. We also know that the closer you live to roads, the more symptoms of hayfever you have. But separating out the different factors was hard. We didn't really know what was going on. What we can say is that having less allergies is highly connected to having a completely different lifestyle.'

It is certainly clear that the less developed countries have much lower rates of allergies. In 1996, the worldwide ISAAC study found an 11.5 per cent annual average prevalence of self-reported asthma symptoms in children aged between thirteen and fourteen across Europe. However, there were huge differences between countries. The rate ranged from 2.6–4.4 per cent in Albania, Romania, Georgia, Greece and the Russian Federation, to 29.1–32.2 per cent in Ireland and the United Kingdom.

Vaccines

There are many people who fear vaccination, particularly for their children. Some think that the immune system can be 'overloaded' by vaccines and that this can contribute to many other conditions, including autism. The 'overloading' theory has no scientific basis at all and although it is widely discredited by scientists, it is still a popular belief.

Could it be that vaccines might actually play a beneficial role in allergy protection? An interesting British study published in 1997 looked at 867 Japanese children who were given the tuberculosis (TB) vaccine at the ages of six and twelve. Those who received the vaccine were three times less likely to develop allergies than those who didn't receive it. This may be because the TB vaccine is made from a weakened version of the *Tuberculosis mycobacterium* and that this prompts a very strong response from the TH1 cells.

However, the story isn't so simple. A further study carried out in Finland on children and young adults who were also given the TB vaccine found that although there was a reduction in allergies among girls and women, there was a marked increase in asthma among boys and men. The overall interpretation is that BCG vaccination doesn't really have a major role to play in determining atopy.

However, scientists were interested because the soil in everyone's garden is full of organisms known as mycobacteria (the kind of organisms that make up the TB vaccine). Getting a bit of dirt on your hands and legs allows the skin to absorb some of them and challenge the immune system. Rolling about in the dirt is not only fun for children, but it may also play a big protective role later in life.

In the 1990s, there was a lot of concern about the whooping cough vaccine, pertussis, after one study suggested that it made more children prone to allergies. A British GP in Oxfordshire had reported seeing an increase in asthma among the children in his practice who had been vaccinated. A further study in New Zealand, dealing with relatively small numbers of children, reported the same thing. But further research did not replicate these findings and one large study in particular, published in the *British Medical Journal* in 1999, found that there was no significant difference in the rate of early wheezing among children who'd been vaccinated in the first six months of life. Doctors also found that when there was a huge loss of public confidence in the whooping cough vaccine in Britain, back in the 1970s, there was no drop off in the number of children with asthma. So it seems very unlikely that the pertussis vaccine is leaving children more at risk from allergies.

Use of antibiotics

Antibiotics are wonderful inventions, as they enable us to defeat bacteria that can be life-threatening. However, some experts believe that the increasing use of antibiotics could be linked to the rising rate of allergies. By upsetting the body's normal balance of microbes that line the gut, antibiotics may prevent our immune system from distinguishing between harmless chemicals and real attacks. It seems that the many millions of microbes which reside in the intestines, known as the gut flora, really work as part of the immune system.

Gary Huffnagle at the University of Michigan in the USA has conducted experiments in mice to show that upsetting the gut flora can provoke an allergic response. His team gave mice a course of antibiotics before feeding some of them with a yeast which is commonly found on human skin. With the natural gut bacteria suppressed by the drugs, the yeast became established in the mouse, with no side effects. Over the course of the following two weeks, the researchers treated all the mice with spores from a common fungus. Again, this does not cause disease, but fungal spores can trigger allergies in people.

The mice whose gut flora had been manipulated experienced a much higher immune response to the spores, suggesting that changes to the collection of microbes in people's guts following antibiotic treatment might also make them more susceptible to allergies. 'Suddenly, your ability to ignore a mould spore has gone,' Huffnagle told the *New Scientist* magazine. He speculates that our gut bacteria are somehow involved in 'training' the immune system to ignore harmless molecules that wind up in our stomach. Precisely how they do this is a mystery, though.

These findings reinforce the message that antibiotics should be used only when absolutely necessary. Some doctors also believe that patients who have just finished antibiotic treatment should also receive probiotic tablets containing 'good' bacteria to restore the balance of healthy gut flora. Eating foods such as raw fruit and vegetables will also help. As Huffnagle points out: 'Once you are done with the antibiotics you are not finished. You need to recover from the treatment itself.'

No one should doubt the misery allergies can cause when they become severe. In Britain, as in other developed countries, there has been a sharp increase in the number of people being admitted to hospital because of severe reactions. A study published in the British Medical Journal in 2004 showed that hospital admissions more than trebled over eleven years. In 1990, 1,960 people were admitted to hospital because of allergic reactions. By 2001, this figure had increased to 6,752. A quarter of them were admitted for anaphylaxis – a sudden, severe and potentially life-threatening reaction, which can cause dangerous swelling of the lips or face and lead to breathing problems (see page 178). Another 18 per cent were admitted for food allergies, with the remaining 17 per cent admitted for angio-oedema – deep swelling underneath the skin, often around the eyes and lips, and sometimes on hands and feet.

John Foreman, Professor of Immunopharmacology at University College London, says scientists are unsure why more people are suffering allergic reactions. 'Nobody really knows why allergies are increasing. There is evidence that there has been an increase in allergic asthma, which is the principal cause of hospital admissions for allergies in the last decade or two. But nobody really knows why this is. One idea is the so-called "muck theory", that children are not as exposed to soil organisms as they used to be and this leaves them more prone to allergies. This is controversial but it is the only idea that I know of that may explain the increase.'

How allergies affect the UK

- Allergic disease affects around one in three of the population.

- The UK has one of the highest rates in the world. In any one year, 12 million people (one fifth of the population) will seek treatment for an allergy.

- 10 per cent of children and adults under the age of forty have two or more atopic disorders.

- The allergies are becoming more severe. Hospital admissions caused by patients suffering anaphylactic shock increased sevenfold in the last decade. Admissions for food allergy reactions increased fivefold.

- Allergies cost the National Health Service an estimated £900m a year, mostly through the prescribed treatments given by GPs.

- 6 per cent of all consultations with the family doctor are about allergies.

- The most common allergies are hayfever, asthma and eczema.

- A survey of 27,500 children carried out in 1999 showed that 20 per cent were reported to have had asthma in the previous year, 18 per cent had hayfever and 16 per cent eczema.

Figures taken from the Royal College of Physicians' report *Allergy: The Unmet Need*, produced in June 2003.

Conclusion

Is our phobia about germs leading us unwittingly into a world where allergies can thrive? Microbes in the soil, bacteria in our gut, the air pollution all around us – all of these invisible substances seem to be somehow implicated in the soaring rates of atopic conditions. The truth is that we don't yet know what it is that causes allergies. However, David Strachan's hygiene hypothesis – or the 'muck theory' as it is also known – seems to come closest to explaining why a society such as the former East Germany that leaves behind an agricultural lifestyle can end up taking on a different kind of problem. As more countries such as Romania join the EU, we might expect to see their 'allergy profile' change in a similar fashion. Also, what about the Melanesian people in the Torres Straits, seeing so many children struggling with asthma attacks? It seems that no corner of the globe is free from the scourge of allergies, even one as seemingly idyllic as theirs.

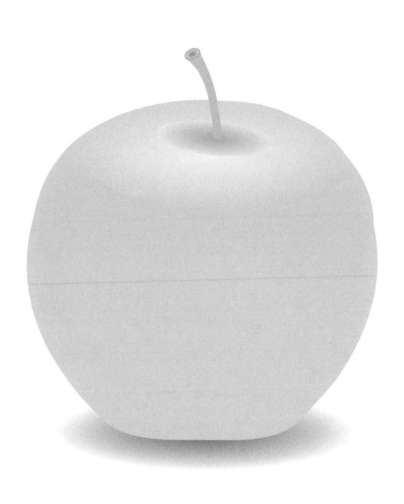

CHAPTER THREE
PREVENTING ALLERGIES

One of the most challenging fields in science right now is the area of allergy prevention. Ever since David Strachan put forward his hygiene hypothesis in 1989 (see page 32), suggesting that perhaps our modern lifestyles and penchant for cleanliness might be unwittingly causing the rise in allergic conditions, there have been many attempts to understand which factors are triggering these responses.

The rather depressing truth is that we still don't know the real causative agents behind allergies. There are a number of suspicious elements that we can point to, such as particular foods and environmental factors such as house-dust mites. Genetics, of course, is hugely important, and the parents' predisposition to allergies is the single best predictor of whether a child will develop them. But this chapter looks at the many different elements which appear to play some kind of contributory role in hypersensitisation. It should be said from the outset that there is no one factor which is going to give you or your child protection from allergies such as asthma, eczema or hayfever.

A friend of mine asked me recently: 'If I could find something that would mean my child didn't have to go through the sneezing and muzzy headedness that I have to endure every June when the pollen count rockets up, then I would gladly pay for it.' Unfortunately, it's not that simple. Many parents want to know, quite rightly, if they can prevent their child from developing allergies, such as asthma or hayfever, which they have themselves. At a time when the incidence of these conditions is rising sharply, it's only natural to want to lower that risk for the next generation.

If you know that at least one of the parents has an allergy, then the question becomes even more relevant and it's a good idea to try and lessen that risk for the offspring by adopting a very healthy lifestyle.

I've set out below the different steps you can take from before birth into adulthood to try and limit the chances of your child becoming hypersensitive to everyday substances.

44

Before the baby is born

While the baby is in the womb it absorbs all the nutrients coming from the mother through the placenta. What the mother eats is generally what is taken in by the baby. That is why having a balanced diet, including plenty of fruit and vegetables and not overeating, will benefit the unborn child. A lot of women are told they can eat what they like during pregnancy, but actually that is probably not the right advice – they should eat healthily. The question of whether pregnant women should eat peanuts during pregnancy has still not been properly answered, but many women do avoid eating them in case they increase the risk of an allergy. Following a more restricted diet, however, is not a good idea – and there's no research to suggest that giving up dairy products, for example, will save your child from any kind of allergy later on.

The single most important step that a pregnant mother can take for her baby is to give up smoking and it's so vital that it cannot be over-emphasised enough. The body has a system for filtering out some of the more harmful chemicals, but others get through. Cigarette smoke, for example, which contains more than fifty different toxins, will reach the baby. It reduces the body's ability to deliver oxygen to the foetus because of the presence of carbon monoxide, cyanide and some hydrocarbons. Apart from being the single biggest risk factor known to stunt the growth of babies, it is linked to allergies, particularly asthma, because it increases the amount of the allergy antibody, IgE, in the body. The number one priority has to be to quit the habit, hard as that is. There are now some very good helplines which offer the best advice, and constant professional support.

The date of birth

Babies born in winter are less likely to develop asthma than those born in the summer months of June to August. This is probably because summer babies will be exposed to the grass pollen floating around. For British children, the highest risks of hayfever appear to be if they are born in April or May, as they will be tiny infants just as the pollen appears in June. Planning the date of the birth, however, is not always that easy… Babies tend to be conceived on their own timescale!

Pets

Parents are often very wary of having pets when a new baby comes into the house. But studies have suggested that children who are exposed to two or more cats and dogs in their first year of life may have a reduced risk of allergy (see also pages 33–34).

Research also indicates that it could lead to boys having a better lung function, for reasons that are still not fully understood. A study, carried out by scientists at the Medical College of Georgia in Augusta, USA and the Henry Ford Health System in Detroit, Michigan, USA looked at 473 children – 241 girls and 232 boys – some of whom had pets up to about the age of seven years old. It tested for atopy – including allergic reaction, lung function and bronchial function – each year. A questionnaire when the children were one year old detailed whether or not they had pets. Concentrations of dust-mite allergens in bedrooms were measured at two years of age.

It was found that those children who had been exposed to pets had half the number of positive skin tests to all the allergens compared to those who had not been exposed. The researchers said that the link was still true when results were adjusted for gender, birth order, parental asthma and smoking, and dust-mite allergen levels. In boys only, it was found that having two or more pets was linked to lower levels of IgE (see page 18), which is linked to hypersensitivity reactions, and better lung function.

However, pets should still not be welcomed into the home if a child or adult has already been diagnosed as asthmatic, since they can exacerbate the condition.

Breastfeeding and diet

The way in which children are fed in their early years may have a considerable impact on the subsequent development of asthma and allergies, according to recent reports.

The Global Allergy and Asthma European Network (GA2LEN), a consortium of European research centres, has started to provide new insights into the role that diet may play in the development of allergies, especially in children.

It concludes that the significant changes in European diets over the past twenty to forty years may have contributed to the increased incidence of allergic diseases.

These experts looked at more than twenty nutrients and defined areas that they think demand further research. They were able to come to some conclusions on three areas – breastfeeding, early diet and probiotics.

The group is headed by Philip Calder, professor of human nutrition at the University of Southampton in the UK. He is working with others to embark on a huge study that will analyse in great detail the diets of children and adults and then compare that data to the development of allergies years later. 'At the moment, there are these three areas that we know have a protective influence against allergies – breastfeeding, healthy early diet and probiotics,' explains Professor Calder. 'But there are many other areas we need to study, and the whole field is very controversial.

'We have looked at antioxidants, for example, which are the good nutrients contained in fruit and vegetables. It seems that a diet which is lacking in antioxidants somehow sets up the immune system to go down the path of over-sensitisation. In some countries, such as the UK, the intake of fruit and veg is slowly rising, but it still isn't nearly enough and most people don't eat the recommended five portions a day.'

Like others, he does not believe that allergies are caused by a poor diet but rather that eating badly is one of several factors which heighten the risk of people becoming allergic. 'There are many other factors, such as your genetics and whether you live in a house filled with cigarette smoke, but we need to get a much better understanding of how our nutrition from our earliest years interacts with the immune system.'

These are the three areas that Calder's team reported on, where there was solid evidence of a protective effect against allergies:

- **Breastfeeding** Breastfeeding alone, without resorting to bottled milk, in the first four months of life is known to be very beneficial for many reasons. When it comes to atopy, it appears to protect the child from a lactose allergy until they are at least eighteen months old and reduces the likelihood of a skin allergy (contact dermatitis) until the age of three. The news is even better when it comes to reducing the risk of a recurrent wheeze and possibly asthma – breastfeeding lowers that risk until the child is six years old. However, the longer term effects of breastfeeding on allergic outcomes are not known and experts say they need further investigation. If both parents are known to be allergic themselves, then breastfeeding is particularly beneficial. But a mother who is finding breastfeeding really hard and may have to use a formula, should not feel guilty for doing so. The question then becomes one of whether she should use the normal formula milks, which are based on cow's milk, or opt for one that is lactose-free. These do appear to protect against eczema and other skin allergies until the child is four years old, and may be safer for an infant whose parents are known to have allergies. Consult your GP for more advice.

- **Healthy early diet** Some components of an infant's diet may have a protective effect too, such as antioxidants found in fruit and vegetables. However, it is currently difficult to point to clear-cut evidence as a lot of the research conducted to date has not been systematic in its approach. The GA2LEN report did suggest that antioxidants such as vitamin C, E and the mineral selenium, which come mainly from fruit and vegetables, do seem to be protective. However reducing your salt intake, increasing magnesium intake and eating apples in particular appears to help some asthmatics.

- **Probiotics** The role of probiotics and prebiotics in the diet is promising. A study has recently shown that they can help reduce the risk of atopic disease by producing changes in the bacteria in the gut that stimulate the immune system.

But what are they, exactly? A probiotic is a dietary supplement which contains beneficial bacteria or yeast, with the most common kinds being lactic acid bacteria, known as LAB. A prebiotic is a food that promotes the growth of certain bacteria in the intestines. What they essentially do is replace the flora or bacteria in the gut with favourable species. It's not a permanent solution, so the probiotics have to be taken every day. There is some suggestion that they can help with eczema and for those with irritable bowel syndrome, but as yet the jury is still out. Professor David Strachan, who founded the hygiene hypothesis (see Chapter Two) is not fully convinced of their benefits and wants to see more research carried out on them before they are widely prescribed.

The balance of fatty acids

In the 1970s, many households began switching from butter to margarine. It was marketed as healthier than butter, because it contained less cholesterol and fewer calories.

But could margarine now be linked to the rise in allergies? The problem all comes down to the balance of fatty acids. Margarine is rich in the essential fatty acid (EFA) Omega 6, but the body also needs to have a certain amount of another EFA ,Omega 3, which mainly comes from oily fish. If the Omega 6 dominates, it can produce a chemical known as prostaglandin E2, which drives the production of the allergy antibody IgE (see page 18).

In this case, it might make sense to give children extra Omega 3 capsules to diminish the chances of having an allergy. It is already known that people who are atopic tend to have lower Omega 3 levels. According to Professor Calder, it is too early to answer this question as studies are so far inconclusive. However, taking an Omega 3 capsule each day does no harm and, since children in many western countries eat very little oily fish, it may be a good idea anyway, because the essential fatty acid has been shown to help brain development and concentration levels.

Protecting against peanut allergy

There is enormous uncertainty over how to avoid a peanut allergy, one of the most serious allergies which can produce a life-threatening anaphylactic response (see p178). In December 2006, scientists in London launched a major study to try and see how parents could reduce the risks of the allergy for their children. The seven-year trial, run by Professor Gideon Lack at King's

College London, will look at whether giving a baby peanut products either increases or decreases the chance of them developing a peanut aversion. 'Recent evidence suggests that children who eat peanut snacks early in life may be protected against peanut allergy, in contrast with previous studies that have suggested the opposite,' says Professor Lack. 'Our study findings may result in a change in public health policy to prevent food allergies and will enable scientists to identify treatment targets to try to develop cures.'

The current advice for parents is that if there is a family history of allergies, whether or not it includes a nut allergy, they should avoid feeding children peanut products before the age of three.

Unpasteurised milk

One of the more intriguing findings of a recent study came about almost by accident. When researchers from the University of London went up to Shropshire to look at the diet and lifestyles of young children in the county, they wanted to compare the lives of those in the rural areas, living on farms, and those in the towns. It has been known for some time that children growing up on a farm are somehow protected from allergies. Studies in Switzerland and Scandinavia have shown this, but no one has pinned down exactly why this is so.

Dirt in the farmyard, touching animals, breathing in stable dust – these were all possible factors put under the spotlight. But what the researchers had not expected was the discovery that drinking unpasteurised milk is somehow linked to not developing asthma, hayfever or eczema later in life.

The study, published in the *Journal of Allergy, Asthma and Immunology* in August 2006, took many people by surprise. For it showed that just a couple of glasses of 'raw' milk a week reduced a child's chances of developing eczema by almost 40 per cent and hayfever by 10 per cent. Blood samples showed raw milk drinkers had 60 per cent lower levels of the antibody IgE.

Researchers believe raw milk contains bacteria that help to prime the immune system. 'It could be that even relatively infrequent exposure to unpasteurised milk is sufficient to have a protective effect,' the researchers concluded.

However, the problem is that this milk is also a source of bacteria that can be toxic. It is for this reason that any unpasteurised milk now sold in England and

Wales has to bear a label clearly spelling out the risk. Despite the study's findings, some experts are warning parents that any benefits are still far outweighed by the chances of their child becoming infected with organisms such as E. coli and campylobacter, two of the main food-poisoning bugs. David Strachan, the man who founded the hygiene hypothesis (see Chapter Two, The Rise in Allergies) was involved in the Shropshire study, and agrees that it is hard to recommend that parents switch to unpasteurised milk. 'If the official advice was suddenly to drink unpasteurised milk, then you couldn't issue that without knowing what the adverse effects might be. What we'd like to do is find out if there is something innocuous within the milk that could provide the basis for a treatment.'

Oils and creams

It's probably the last thing you would think of, but mothers should be careful of which lotions and creams they use to soothe their baby's skin or any kind of rash in case it triggers a reaction that leads to food allergy months later.

A large study carried out by a team from Imperial College in London followed nearly 14,000 children from the womb through to the age of six. Researchers compared potential predisposing factors to peanut allergy in children who developed the sensitivity with those who didn't. They found that forty nine of those who developed peanut allergy had showed the characteristic weals, flushing and hives if they had been first exposed to peanuts by the age of two. Further investigation by the researchers uncovered that many of these children had already had skin contact with creams and oils containing anywhere from 0.3 per cent to 100 per cent peanut oil.

Peanuts are one of the most common foods to trigger allergic responses and in the USA alone, some 1.5 million people have a demonstrated sensitivity to the proteins in this food. But the allergy isn't produced after the first exposure to peanuts. There have to be several early encounters, during which those who are susceptible start to create antibodies to the protein contained in the legume. And it doesn't have to be from food. A study, published in the *New England Journal of Medicine* pointed out that some of the creams containing peanut oil had been marketed as treatments for nappy rash, and a few were targeted to treat scaly scalps. In this study, children whose skin had been exposed to such products were 6.8 times as likely to develop peanut allergy compared with those exposed only to peanut-free products.

Many cosmetics, body lotions, hydrating creams and soaps do contain peanut oils, nut oils and soy oils, according to Lack, who now runs an allergy clinic at Guy's and St Thomas' Hospital, London. 'Although not directly prescribed for use on infant skin,' he notes, 'it's not uncommon for mothers to apply these products on their babies – because these preparations are marketed as benign and good for the skin.

51

The fascinating thing, Lack says, was the apparent lack of risk from babies' possibly absorbing any of the cream mothers put on their breasts, which may contain peanut oil. 'Children who are suckling the breast would ingest these oils that mothers had been applying to their chapped nipples,' he observes, 'and would therefore seem to face an elevated risk of allergy.'

But his data showed there was the same rate of usage of these creams containing peanut oil in the mothers of children who did and those who didn't develop peanut allergy. Moreover, mothers of children with peanut allergy hadn't consumed more of the legumes during pregnancy or lactation than had other mothers.

One theory is that because the baby is absorbing the protein through the skin, the substance isn't going through the intestines and therefore the normal immune process isn't working. It could be the case that exposures during childhood to tiny amounts of proteins can give you a low dose which is actually worse than a high-dose exposure. The new British study found that certain additional factors appeared to distinguish some of the children who developed peanut allergy. For instance, they were, as a group, 2.6 times as likely as the other youngsters to have a history of rashes over joints and skin creases and five times as likely to have experienced oozing, crusted rashes. Both symptoms may show that these children have a heightened immune sensitivity to begin with.

Antibiotics

When you have an infection, doctors sometimes write a prescription for antibiotics, a class of drugs which kill off the harmful bacteria. For many years, antibiotics have been over-prescribed around the world, leading to a dangerous build up of illnesses which become resistant to these drugs. Many countries, including Britain, are now trying to cut back on prescription, so doctors won't hand them out unless they feel there is a good reason for patients to have them, for example, for chest and ear infections or after surgery, in order to prevent really dangerous infections from taking hold.

But some believe that the increasing prevalence of allergies may be linked to antibiotic use. As the work on food intolerance shows (see page 124) there is a suspicion that people who have been on a prolonged course of antibiotics are then more likely to develop gut problems which can cause an intolerance to a common food group.

There is also emerging evidence that asthma may be exacerbated by antibiotics. A recent British study found that if children were given antibiotics before the age of two, they had an increased risk of asthma later in childhood. The risk seems to be greater for some antibiotics than others – erythromycin seems to be worse, for example, than penicillin. If your child does have to have a course of these drugs, talk it through with your doctor. If he or she feels that the infection needs to be controlled with antibiotics, do follow the medical advice, rather than risk the illness getting worse.

Cleanliness

We come back again to the hygiene hypothesis, outlined in Chapter Two (page 32). For so many parents, keeping the house clean and tidy and making sure the children don't become grubby little monsters is all-important. But it may not be the right strategy for protecting them against allergies.

The truth is that children who are kept 'too clean' do run a higher risk of developing asthma. One study showed that having two baths a day and washing the hands five times a day means the risk of having asthma is increased by 25 per cent, nearly twice as high as those children who only have a bath every two days. Playing in the mud is extremely important. The soil contains all sorts of fungi and bacteria which challenge the young immune system and enable the child to be exposed to them. Just being outside is extremely good too. In particular, it keeps the airways healthy and strengthens the muscles around the lungs and the trachea. It also keeps the child fit and less likely to become overweight, which in itself is a risk factor for an allergy in later years.

The home

House-dust mites are tiny insects about 0.3mm long and are transparent, so they can only be seen with a microscope. They live in the dust that builds up around the house, in carpets, bedding, beds, soft furnishings and soft toys. Up to 85 per cent of people with allergic asthma are sensitive to house-dust mites and their droppings.

It seems to make sense that in order to prevent over-sensitisation to these mites from building up, you should reduce the numbers of them sharing your home with you. An entire science now lies behind eliminating these creatures, but it doesn't mean that you have to spend a fortune. The numbers can be reduced significantly by using barrier covers on beds and bedding, hot washing bedding weekly, regular vacuuming and damp dusting surfaces daily (see Chapter Twelve, Your Home, for more information).

If you are redecorating the home, you could give serious consideration to have wooden or lino floors with rugs instead of a carpet. In the 1950s, every good housewife would take out the rug once a week into the garden and beat it to get rid of the dust and dirt. This is probably a lot better than vacuuming, which can just scatter mites and allergens all over the place. Washing curtains regularly or replacing them with blinds and reducing humidity levels also helps. Central heating isn't great because it means there is little circulation of the air.

Lowering the risk when you're an adult

There is no foolproof way that you can avoid getting an allergy, but there are certainly habits you can adopt to help you minimise the risk. Giving up smoking has to be one of the most effective ways of clearing the airways and preventing allergies. And as exercise helps children, it also helps adults. We know that being overweight or obese does increase the chances of you becoming allergic, so keeping the weight off is very important.

There are also new areas which scientists are now investigating. One of them is what you can do to protect the lower and upper airways from inflammation, which occurs as part of the body's response against allergens such as pollen or house-dust mites. Aspirin hit the headlines in January 2007, when a large US study of 22,000 people found that the painkiller reduced the risk of being diagnosed asthmatic by as much as 22 per cent, a very significant amount. The results were not expected – in fact, the scientists had done the study in order to understand whether aspirin could reduce the risk of a heart attack.

In addition to helping to protect the heart, they also found that people taking a low-dose aspirin every other day also considerably lowered their risk of receiving an asthma diagnosis.

However, it cannot be said that aspirin is a cure-all that reduces the severity of asthma once it's been diagnosed. The painkiller can actually cause severe bronchospasm in some patients who have the condition, since around one in five asthmatics are at risk of having a severe reaction to the drug (see Chapter Five, Asthma, p86).

PART TWO
THE ALLERGIES

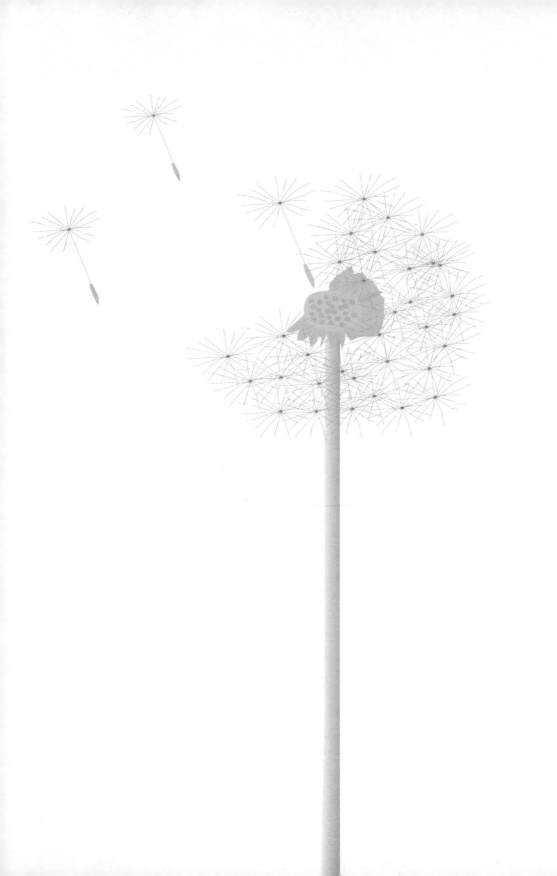

CHAPTER FOUR
HAYFEVER

Something untoward was picked up by the weather satellites in May 2006. A giant yellow pollen cloud could be seen drifting from the forests of Denmark and Scandinavia across the North Sea to England. The fine grains were blown across Europe, with the images of the cloud being captured on satellite photographs. The size and intensity of this phenomenon was unprecedented – and so was its effect, as it left thousands of people across Europe with the misery of watering eyes and runny noses weeks before the usual peak of the hayfever season. Experts saw it as a harbinger of things to come. They warned that as the climate continues to warm up, so the pollen seasons are lengthening with trees and grasses flowering earlier. Also, changes in the atmosphere itself – with greater levels of carbon dioxide present – could result in an increase in pollen production.

On one Sunday that May, Denmark recorded its highest pollen count level ever – a record 4,381 grains of pollen per cubic metre of air, while Vienna recorded 2,500pcm. In England, the levels reached over 1,000pcm, which was certainly cause for concern as 80pcm is considered high.

One of those who is closely watching the situation is Professor Jean Emberlin, Director of the National Pollen and Aerobiology Research Unit in England. 'There are several aspects to the problem,' she told reporters at the end of 2006. 'Firstly, the pollen season for trees is coming earlier with climate changes. In the UK, over the last thirty years, the tree pollen season has got earlier by five days per decade. Secondly, the grass pollen season is tending to go on longer in the summer. Twenty years ago, it was probably finished by the end of July. However, these days, it often goes on until the first or second week of August and this is reflected in GP consultation rates for hayfever.

Thirdly, there has been a trend in the last thirty years for the effects of grass pollen to become more severe.' She explained that when plants are put under 'stress' by rising temperatures, they tend to produce more protein on the pollen grain to increase their chances of production. It is this protein which causes the immune reaction, so the same amount of pollen has a more pronounced effect. As Professor Emberlin put it: 'Quite a lot of factors are all pressing towards a scenario where we have an increasing allergenic load.'

60

Hayfever is the most common allergy in Western countries, affecting around 15 per cent of the population. In the UK, the rates have soared and it is staggering to think that some 26 per cent of the population now suffer from it, usually for around two to three months each year. The condition, also known as seasonal allergic rhinitis, is often thought of as a minor ailment whereas, in reality, the constant tiredness and sneezing that is all part of the condition can have a very real impact on peoples' lives. Around the globe, some $20 billion is spent on hayfever each year, a figure which includes medication, time off work, and physician consultations. Despite this, many patients are still very bad at getting themselves the treatment they need.

What is hayfever?

Put at its most simple, hayfever is an acute allergic reaction to airborne particles which get into your nose, throat and upper respiratory passages, causing the body to produce antibodies and release chemicals known as histamines.

We all know when the hayfever season is upon us because, even if you're not a sufferer, you are surrounded by people who are sneezing and rubbing their eyes. The symptoms may seem no more than that of a common cold to those who don't suffer, but the allergy can be really debilitating and can stop people from working productively. For children, it can be a nightmare especially if they have exams coming up because the condition makes them feel woozy and tired, and there is evidence that it affects their ability to think clearly during these months. It's also embarrassing to have red, watery eyes and a streaming nose every time you step outside to enjoy the sun.

The most common allergens causing hayfever are grass pollen and pollen from trees such as elder, elm, hazel and especially birch. In the autumn, hayfever can be triggered by the pollen from mugwort and plants such as chrysanthemum (see page 63 for more on this).

There is also the growing threat of hayfever from house-dust mites and fungus spores that come from mould – these often appear in the autumn. This is known as perennial allergic rhinitis, a condition which can occur all year round, rather than just during the spring and summer months.

What causes it?

It all comes down to the workings of the respiratory tract. The nose, the sinuses and the lower airway are lined with a thin mucous membrane, which is covered in tiny hairs (ciliated) containing the mucous glands. It is the sensitivity of that membrane which determines your response to the allergens that reach it.

61

Generally speaking, the microscopic substances, such as pollen, which get into the nose would not normally trigger a problem – the body would simply flush them away. But in those with a hypersensitivity, they cause the body to produce particular antibodies, including IgE, and release histamine. This is a messenger chemical, which can cause several different reactions such as irritating the upper respiratory passages, making them swell and causing the blood vessels to expand. These reactions, in turn, produce the blockage, itching and sneezing in the nose and cause the skin to itch.

What are the symptoms?
- Itchy and watery eyes
- Frequent sneezing, a bunged up or runny nose
- Itching on the roof of the mouth
- Coughing
- Tightening of the throat or chest
- Wheezing or a burning sensation in the throat
- Lethargy
- Loss of concentration

Long-term consequences

If you are a hayfever sufferer, it is important that you avoid the substances that provoke hypersensitivity otherwise you will increase the risk of developing other more serious allergic conditions such as asthma and also sleeping difficulties that can lead to chronic fatigue (because of blocked nasal passages and snoring). When a particle of pollen gets into your nose, it produces sneezing, congestion and a watery discharge. When a piece of house-dust mite hits the lower airway, it can prompt coughing, wheezing or a shortness of breath. But what can happen over time is that you develop a 'nasal hyper reactivity' to these allergens which causes both a nasal blockage in the upper part and sneezing in the lower part. This reaction is caused by the same chemicals – the histamines, prostaglandins, leukotrienes and various chemicals – that were discussed in Chapter One, How Allergies Work.

The good news is that hayfever treatments have improved in recent years, with new ones currently in development. Even though you can't get rid of the allergy itself, the symptoms can be controlled and, for the majority of sufferers, the condition is more of a nuisance than a danger to health.

The links between asthma and hayfever

We tend to think of these two as separate allergies, but doctors are becoming increasingly aware of how closely they are linked. The growth of asthma is now being mirrored in the exponential rise in hayfever which, perhaps, shouldn't come as a surprise. After all, both affect our respiratory tract and appear to have a similar response of coughing and shortness of breath.

There is emerging evidence that hayfever may be a risk factor for the development of asthma and we know that 60 per cent of asthma sufferers also experience similar symptoms such as a blocked or runny nose, sneezing and itchy eyes. A study carried out in 2005 revealed that nearly 50 per cent of asthmatics found that when their rhinitis was active, their asthma symptoms were exacerbated. Most of them suffered from the seasonal form of hayfever rather than the year-long perennial rhinitis. The links between the two may seem fairly depressing, but on the other hand it does allow the suggestion that by treating hayfever properly as soon as it appears, asthma might actually be avoided.

The hayfever season

Thanks to the rising temperatures experienced across the world in recent years, the pattern of the seasons is changing and with it comes an alteration in the time pollen is released. According to records, 2006 was a particularly bad year because many trees across Europe flowered early. In the UK, the hayfever season starts as early as January with the release of certain pollens, peaks between the first half of June until mid-July because that is when grass releases most of its pollens and can last through until October. Different plants have different times for pollen release. In England:

Early spring – hazel, yew, elm, willow and alder

Mid-spring – birch

End spring to early autumn – common chestnut, weeds such as nettles and dock

Summer – grass pollen

Early autumn – mould spores inside the house, often from bathrooms

Early to mid-autumn – mugwort and hybrids such as chrysanthemum

Diagnosis

Firstly, your doctor needs to confirm that it is definitely hayfever you are suffering from and not some other condition. Secondly, they need to establish which pollen or combination of pollens are causing your allergy. To find out, a skin-prick test (see page 141) is carried out to see how you respond to the various pollens that are around throughout the year. To help the doctor, it may be useful to keep a diary which records when exactly your symptoms are at their worst.

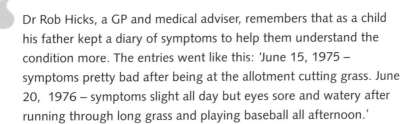

Dr Rob Hicks, a GP and medical adviser, remembers that as a child his father kept a diary of symptoms to help them understand the condition more. The entries went like this: 'June 15, 1975 – symptoms pretty bad after being at the allotment cutting grass. June 20, 1976 – symptoms slight all day but eyes sore and watery after running through long grass and playing baseball all afternoon.'

He recalls: 'Over the years, it soon became apparent which situations were likely to result in me suffering symptoms and what could be done to prevent this. The key to allergy management is to avoid the triggers as best you can but also to know what treatments work for you and to have them ready. Basically, it's about being prepared – as all good cub scouts know.'

Treatment

• Avoidance of pollens

This is sometimes easier said than done, but avoiding the allergen that is causing your symptoms is very important and can make a big difference to your life. Here are some useful tips:

- If the pollen count is high, try to stay indoors and keep away from grassy areas.

- Avoid parks, fields and walking through long grass.

- Don't let the pollen indoors. Drying clothes inside rather than on the washing line can help because the pollen can be carried inside on the laundry. It may sound rather drastic, but keeping a change of clothes just inside the door so that you can change as soon as you come inside can really help reduce the risk. The clothes you've worn outside should then be put into a bag and washed as soon as possible to remove any traces of pollen. It's also a good idea to have a bath or shower to wash off any pollen that may be sticking to your hair or clothes.

- Doors and windows should be kept closed to stop pollen from drifting in. You can even put a sheet over the bed so that any dust that comes in doesn't get on your pillow. Vacuum every couple of days to pick up any stray pollen.

- Pets can also carry pollen inside. Try to wipe them down when they come into the house as they will be carrying it in their fur. Don't let pets get close to your face and always wash your hands after stroking a pet.

- Wear wrap-around sunglasses. Not only are they cool, but they will also prevent allergens getting into the corner of your eyes. Another trick is to apply some kind of barrier cream such as petroleum jelly to the insides of your nostrils. This will trap the pollen before it can get inside the nose and trigger your symptoms. Remember that you will need to reapply it every couple of hours or so.

- When you're out driving, keep car windows closed.

- Investigate the possibility of fitting your car with a pollen filter to keep pollen out.

Pollen forecasts

Pollen counts or forecasts are now given regularly in newspapers, radio and on websites to warn people how much pollen is in the air. It's measured in grains of pollen per square metre of air (pcm) based on the average collected over a 24-hour period.

Most forecasts will say whether the count is low, moderate, high or very high on a daily basis. On high days, it's best to remain indoors as much as possible. If you do have to go out, then try to do so during the middle of the day, because that is when the pollen is high in the atmosphere. The pollen is released early morning, so you'll be vulnerable at that stage, between 5am and 10am, and again during the later afternoon and early evening, when the air cools, and the pollen falls back down to earth.

• Medications

Antihistamines

If avoidance is not possible or does not relieve symptoms, additional treatment is needed. Many patients respond to antihistamines, a very widely used class of drugs. These substances combat the histamine that has been released during an allergic reaction, by blocking the action of the histamine on the body.

Antihistamines don't stop the formation of histamine and nor do they stop the conflict between the IgE antibody and the allergen. What they do is protect the body's tissues from the fallout of the allergic reaction. The drugs have been around for forty years and have a very good safety record, but side effects can include sleepiness and a dry mouth.

It's now possible in most countries to buy over-the-counter antihistamines and many people prefer to take them as a tablet or capsule. For children, they are available as syrups or in a sugar-free form. These drugs can also be found as nasal sprays or eye drops.

The older antihistamines, such as Atarax, Piriton (chlorphenamine), Tavegil and Optimine, can induce sleepiness, as well as poor co-ordination. That may or may not be a problem for a patient – it really depends on the kind of work they are doing during the day. The newer variants such as Clarityn, Semprex, Mizollen and Terfenadine are non-sedating and do not cause drowsiness. Some of these need prescriptions and others don't. It's important to talk through your symptoms with your doctor and find the drug that works for you. It is also important to discuss the other possible side effects that very occasionally occur (such as urine retention in men, or a fast heart rate).

Two of the newer antihistamines (Terfenadine and Astemizole, brand names Hismanal and Pollen-eze) have, on rare occasions, had life-threatening or fatal side effects. When overdosed or combined with one of a small number of other medicines, or in people with certain kinds of heart trouble, they have been known to cause the heart to beat in an abnormal way, and among the vast numbers of people who have taken the drug, a small number have died. Terfenadine is available in Britain on prescription only and Astemizole has been withdrawn from use in the UK. A new medicine called Telfast in Britain (Allegra in the USA), whose official name is Fexofenadine, is the successor to Terfenadine.

Antihistamines can also be administered via a nasal spray. Levocabastine nasal spray is a spray that contains an antihistamine. Instead of taking the medicine orally, you simply breathe it in through the nose. Its brand name is Livostin.

Decongestants

These help control allergy symptoms (but not the causes) by shrinking the swollen membranes in the nose and making it easier to breathe. They can be taken orally or by nasal spray, but should not be used for longer than five days without the advice of a doctor and usually only when accompanied by a nasal steroid (see below). This is because they often cause a rebound effect if taken for too long a period. A rebound effect is the worsening of symptoms when a drug is discontinued and is a result of a tissue dependence on the medication. Common decongestants (and their brand names) are pseudoephedrine pills (Sudafed), oxymetazoline (Vicks Sinex), phenylephrine (Fenox) and xylometazoline (Otrivine, Sudafed Nasal Spray).

The decongestant cromolyn is a prescription medicine which inhibits the mast cells, one of the key cell types involved in the allergic reaction and blocks the release of histamine. It is available as a nasal spray or eye drops. The over-the-counter form of this medication is the nasal spray Nasalcrom, available in some countries. It has to be used well in advance of the hayfever season, because the effects take approximately two weeks to be felt. It's a safe drug and can be used for long-term treatment.

Steroid nasal sprays and eye drops

Brand names include Flixonase and Beconase which can be bought over the counter, and Vancenase, Nasonex and Nasalide which are only available on prescription. These can effectively limit reactions to allergens by reducing the inflammation which causes the sneezing and runny nose. It takes several days for a steroid nasal spray to build up to its full effect and it must be taken every day during the hayfever season in order for it to be effective. Typical side effects are generally minor and can include an unpleasant smell or taste, nosebleeds and irritation inside the nose. Applying a tiny amount of petroleum jelly inside your nose before using a nasal steroid can help counteract this.

Alternatively, you may prefer to use a salt water saline nose spray which works by helping to clean out allergens caught in the nasal passages and keeping the passages moist.

Some of the medicines mentioned also come in eye-drop form to relieve allergy-related eye problems. Steroid eye drops are sometimes given for severe inflammation of the eye during the hayfever season, However, their use can increase your risk of getting an eye infection, so they should only be used under medical supervision.

Leukotriene blockers

This newer class of medicines is normally used for asthma sufferers (see page 85). However, they can be used with antihistamines to relieve symptoms of hayfever by reducing the swelling inside the nose and making it easier to breathe. Two common prescription-only leukotriene blockers (and their brand names) are montelukast (Singulair) and zafirlukast (Accolate). They help some patients to sneeze less frequently and their noses also feel less itchy.

Your doctor may recommend the use of one of these sprays along with an antihistamine to combat your symptoms.

• Immunotherapy

For years, scientists have talked about immunotherapy as the perfect treatment for hayfever as well as other allergies. This is where the sufferer is given gradually increasing doses of the substance to which they are allergic, such as grass pollen or house-dust mite, so the immune system becomes less sensitive to it and forms natural antibodies that will block future adverse reactions. It is a gradual process which typically takes as long as three to four years and is not always successful.

It is the only treatment which actually involves tackling the underlying disease, rather than the symptoms, but in the UK it has had rather a chequered history. The first clinical report of immunotherapy for allergies appeared in *The Lancet* in 1911, when hayfever sufferers were successfully treated with injections of pollen extracts. Since then, immunotherapy has been adopted in North America and Europe as a treatment for allergic rhinitis, but in the UK its use has been limited, partly due to a ruling by the Committee on the Safety of Medicines (CSM) made in 1986. This stated that immunotherapy must only be given where there is resuscitation equipment available and that all patients must wait an hour after each injection. The requirement for resuscitation equipment ruled out most GP surgeries which effectively put immunotherapy beyond the reach of many allergy sufferers, owing to the shortage of allergy specialists and hospital clinics. The CSM ruling was prompted by a number of deaths due to immunotherapy, caused by patients going into anaphylactic shock (see page 178) after having the treatment. However, almost all of these deaths were due to very basic errors in the way the injections were given and, today, there is very little risk of suffering a bad reaction because safety procedures are now so stringent.

In January 2007, British scientists carried out a review pooling all the data from fifty-one different clinical trials. They were looking at whether injecting a tiny amount of pollen extract just below the skin in people who have hayfever could reduce their symptoms. They concluded that the procedure did work, but needed to be carried out in specialist centres.

A systematic review by The Cochrane Collaboration, an initiative to look at large amounts of data worldwide to assess the impact of treatments, was encouraging. They looked at studies that involved a total of 2,871 patients,

1,645 of whom received an active treatment, while 1,226 received an inactive placebo. The treatment consisted of an average of eighteen injections spread over a range of times from three days to three years. The review concluded that immunotherapy is a safe and valid treatment for patients with hayfever, particularly those who have not responded to other treatments. It reduced symptoms and meant many patients did not need so much medication.

They also found that serious adverse reactions to the therapy had happened in only four patients, one of whom had been given a placebo. Three had an anaphylactic reaction and one had an attack of asthma, but all of them recovered fully.

The future for hayfever sufferers

At the moment, the only immunotherapy available for hayfever sufferers is monthly injections of hayfever vaccine, but in practice very few patients receive them because in countries such as Britain, you have to go to a specialist allergy centre as there is a risk of serious reactions.

Medical researchers are now concentrating on developing different preventative treatments – the Holy Grail for all allergists. The first vaccine pill for hayfever sufferers who are allergic to grass pollen has been launched in twenty-seven countries across Europe, including Britain where it became available in February 2007, promising to bring about a huge reduction in symptoms among sufferers. According to clinical trials, this new pill, Grazax, reduces the symptoms of runny noses and watering eyes more than antihistamines and steroid nasal sprays. And, most importantly, it works for around 30 per cent of patients who cannot get proper relief from the other medications.

The pill, developed by a Danish company, contains small amounts of grass pollen extract and works by 'persuading' the immune system to react in the right way to the allergen. Instead of just working on the symptoms, it tackles the illness itself.

In trials, patients given Grazax reported a 30 per cent reduction in symptoms and a 40 per cent fall in the need for relief medication. 82 per cent of participants said they felt 'better' or 'much better' than in previous years.

Grazax – whose active ingredient is derived from Timothy grass, a common grass – is available on prescription and is taken by placing it under the tongue daily for a minimum of two months before the pollen season starts. A large trial is now underway to see how effective the pills might be in the long term, once patients have stopped taking them.

Stephen Durham, Professor of Allergy and Respiratory Medicine at the Royal Brompton Hospital and Imperial College, London, said: 'The tablet should lead to a much more acceptable form of therapy. It should be targeted at those who do not respond to the usual therapy and must be prescribed by a specialist.'

Many specialists believe that such immunotherapy holds the key to revolutionising the way in which hayfever is treated. As it treats the cause not just the symptoms of the condition, it paves the way for developing preventative measures.

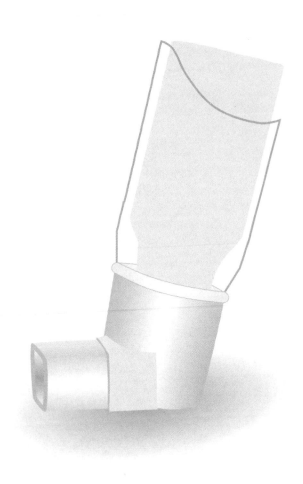

CHAPTER FIVE
ASTHMA

Britain, the United States, Australia and New Zealand all share the unhappy similarity of having the highest asthma rates in the world, with one in every five households having a sufferer – and no one really knows why. The burden that the condition places on both children and adults is considerable and is largely not understood by people who have never experienced it for themselves. In Britain, a child is admitted to hospital with asthma every nineteen minutes and one person dies of it every six hours. If this were a new infectious disease, there would be a public outcry but, because it is a common, chronic condition, we somehow accept it with a shrug of the shoulders.

I have to say that the severity of the condition had not really hit home with me until I began to research the book and talk to affected families. It was then that I realised that despite all the advances in medicine and improvements in management of symptoms, asthma can be the defining experience of one's life. A friend of mine, Diana, led me through the story of her son's asthma, and I began to understand how dramatically it had affected the entire family. Her youngest son, Jack, has mild asthma, but her oldest son, Stephen, who is now seventeen, has suffered badly from it since he was a baby.

 case study ———————————————————————

Stephen had wheezed since he was a baby and by the time he started school, we knew he was asthmatic – just like my father and my sister. It was very hard for him at that stage because he wanted to run around with the other children, but doing so just exacerbated his condition.

'The winter months were awful because he would pick up every virus going and then be very ill. Often, he would have three weeks off school at a time, which affected his education.

'The coughing at night was the worst, and my husband and I would hear this tight little cough and go straight to his bedside. He would be so distressed as the coughing woke him up – too distressed at first to use his inhaler, so we would sit either side of him and try to calm him down, until we could get him to use it. To see your child unable to breathe is a really terrible experience.

'Like many parents, we didn't really appreciate at first that Stephen needed to see a specialist. However, at the age of eleven, he was referred to the Royal Brompton Hospital in London and saw a wonderful doctor who immediately put him on a two-week course of stronger steroids. This definitely helped his asthma but unfortunately it had the side effect of making him very aggressive, very difficult. He certainly seemed to change during that period.

'For the most part, his condition continued improving but he was finding it very hard to go to school. It's difficult to know whether the mood swings he was experiencing were the result of the medication he was on, or because the whole experience had just affected him so much.

'He was making such good progress that during one hospital appointment, the doctors decided to take him off all his medication altogether. A part of me thought fantastic, no more steroids. But a few months later, he got a virus which really laid him low. We went out a few days later for a pizza and I suddenly noticed his throat going in and out like a little pump. He couldn't breathe. He was rushed into hospital, where he spent several days in intensive care. It was a very frightening time.

'He went back on to steroids and his condition slowly improved. It may also have helped that as he grew bigger, his lungs also grew and this improved his condition. Stephen also learned how to take his preventer medication regularly and knows more now about the warning signs so he is now very aware of his condition.

'Stephen is now seventeen, and the condition has really improved. He manages it well and totally by himself but I think it has had a profound effect on our relationship with him and also on his education. Looking back, I find it painful to remember how bad some of those early days were, when I would set up my camp bed in his room, just to ensure that he would make it through the night.'

case study

What is it?

Asthma is a condition that affects the airways – the small tubes that carry air in and out of the lungs. It is a chronic illness that tends to run in families and often begins in childhood but can develop at any age and, in severe cases, can be life-threatening. Even in mild cases, it can be a very debilitating illness which needs careful management at all times. However, by getting to know the individual triggers which prompt the asthma, and taking the appropriate medication, for most people it is a manageable condition.

Within the lungs, there are thousands and thousands of hollow tubes, known as the bronchi and the bronchioles. They look a bit like the branches of a tree and they carry air to and from the tiny air sacs that help us to absorb oxygen and get rid of carbon dioxide. These are what are known as the airways. When a person with asthma comes into contact with something that irritates their airways, the lining of these tubes becomes inflamed. This inflammation causes the lining to swell, narrowing the tubes and making the normal process of breathing harder. At this stage, the airways often start overproducing mucus which can cause them to clog up even further.

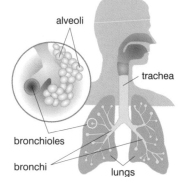

The swollen airways then lead to a sudden, painful tightening of the muscles around the chest, called a bronchospasm. For a sufferer, it can cause great distress and panic as they literally feel they are fighting for every breath. This is what is commonly known as an asthma attack.

A bronchospasm occurs because the cells lining the airways have become oversensitised and are reacting to different triggers or irritants. These are not always allergens, such as pollen, but can be substances that can act on the airway if it is already inflamed such as a cold or viral infection, being in a smoky atmosphere, walking out into cold air or simply feeling extremely anxious. As the airways become more constricted, the air that is already in the lungs doesn't leave at the normal rate, so when the sufferer next inhales, there is still some stale air in the lungs. This increases the pain because the muscles around the chest have to stretch further to accommodate the extra air. At the same time, the sufferer may start to wheeze. This is the sound the air makes when it is travelling through the narrowed airways.

Being in control

For many people with asthma, taking the appropriate medication effectively dampens down the inflammation, keeping symptoms at bay and enabling them to carry on with normal living. However, the big hidden problem for many sufferers is when their condition is not properly managed and they end up having serious and frightening attacks.

According to the charity Asthma UK, more than half of Britain's 5.1 million asthmatics suffer severe symptoms. A report written by the charity in May 2004 concluded that, for thousands of sufferers, there are still no medicines that adequately control their condition. In Scotland, where asthma kills about 100 people each year, the charity said more than 40,000 people were living in constant fear of a fatal attack. In the UK, 1,400 people die a year from the condition, partly because too few were prescribed the newer steroid inhalers (LABAs, see page 82) that would have improved the quality of their treatment.

Surveys also carried out by the charity suggest that some 500,000 asthmatics are afraid their next attack will kill them, while one in six have regular attacks so severe they cannot speak. For some of these patients, effective management could easily improve their quality of life. Many were found not to have essential personal asthma action plans – a written management plan agreed with their doctor or asthma nurse detailing all the information they need regarding medication or worsening of symptoms in order to help them control their condition.

Can asthma be inherited?

Since the 1920s, doctors have known that asthma is passed down in families, suggesting at least some kind of genetic basis to the disease. But in those days, they also believed that there were strong psychological causes; patients were labelled as 'asthmatic types', and often their parents were told they had created the breathing difficulties by making them anxious and stressed.

We now know this not to be the case, although stress does exacerbate the condition. Scientists are still unsure of the nature of our genetic susceptibility to asthma, but several studies recently have suggested that genes may play a stronger role than initially thought. Across the world, different laboratories have uncovered several 'candidate' genes which are linked to asthma – these are genes which are likely to play some kind of role in the development of the allergy.

The problem for science is that asthma is a complex disease, hard to define and hard to study. To some scientists, even the word asthma is outdated because it suggests one disease, rather than allowing them to define all the different forms it can take. Writing in *The Lancet* in 2006, Dr Sally Wenzel of the National Jewish Medical and Research Center in Denver, Colorado, USA, said that asthma should be sub-classified into different types, based on the triggers for the symptoms and its clinical characteristics. But most doctors feel that it is currently impossible to do this, because there isn't yet enough knowledge of the different types.

It is likely that within the next decade there will be far more genetic information available, which will enable us to tease out the relationship between a particular 'allergy' gene and other factors including environmental issues such as cigarette smoking and the role of diet. Pharmaceutical companies talk about a 'genomics revolution' when new medications will be created to target particular genetic flaws but, for the moment, in 2007, that remains a distant hope.

Diagnosis

There is no simple definition of asthma because there are so many different symptoms and characteristics of the disease. However, most people are able to get a diagnosis because GPs tend to know it when they see it. The treatments that are now available are far better at controlling the shortness of breath and the underlying problems it produces than they were twenty years ago, and the risk of death is much lower. But in Britain, there are still many thousands of people who go undiagnosed because they fail to tell the doctor the extent of their symptoms.

Getting a proper diagnosis is crucial. In many European countries, the GP will make the initial diagnosis before referring you to a specialist asthma nurse who will talk to you about coping strategies and managing your condition. In the USA, you may be referred to a paediatrician if you are worried about your child's health.

Before making the diagnosis, your doctor will want to find out more about you or your child's symptoms – what they are, when they happen and how long they have been going on. The next stage is likely to be a lung-function test, which measures how well the air is filling up and emptying in the lungs. For this, a machine known as a spirometer is used. The test is likely to look at peak flow, the maximum speed at which the air leaves your lungs as you exhale. The doctor will also measure the residual volume, the amount of air left in the lungs after you have exhaled, which is measured with a plethysmograph.

• Diagnosing the condition in babies

The number of children who suffer from asthma is increasing and, in Western countries, around 50 per cent of sufferers develop symptoms by the age of two. It is a difficult illness to diagnose in a child because it shares so many symptoms with other conditions and because it's also very difficult to measure with any accuracy how well babies, in particular, are breathing.

One of the conditions which presents many similar symptoms to asthma in young children is bronchiolitis. This is usually caused by a viral infection known as Respiratory Synctial Virus (RSV). The bronchioles, the tiny air passages that lead to the lungs, become swollen and babies can find it hard to breathe as they get filled up with mucus. Scientists know that babies with bronchiolitis are more likely to develop asthma later on, but it's not clear whether the infection can trigger asthma, or whether the baby had an increased risk of developing breathing problems in the first place.

Wheezing is also another difficult area. Babies born prematurely whose lungs are not fully developed, may wheeze but that doesn't necessarily mean they will go on to develop asthma. All parents want a diagnosis as early as possible, but doctors may not want to commit themselves until the child is a little older. An awful lot of babies wheeze as infants and don't develop asthma – probably two-thirds of wheezing infants eventually outgrow it. However, some doctors do like to err on the side of caution and may start to treat the condition as if it is asthma before it is entirely clear to them. This is due to evidence that suggests the early use of medications to control inflammation may prevent any further damage to the lungs.

Warning signs for children

If your child has recurrent wheezing, constant periods of coughing, particularly if they worsen at night, and any other breathing problems, it is important to talk to your doctor. Tell them about any family history of allergies or sinus problems. Also, be honest with them. If you smoke, it is important to let them know because smoking is linked to children's breathing difficulties. There are many children who suffer from persistent coughs which are simply due to their parents' smoking.

79

Identifying the causes

To effectively manage asthma, it is crucial to know what your own particular triggers are. In the case of allergens such as pollen, house-dust mites, pets and so on, a skin-prick test (see page 141) is the best way of identifying which are the culprits. Unfortunately, in Britain, patients don't find it easy to get such a test through the NHS, as there are so few specialist allergy clinics where they are done. Instead, many GPs tend to assume that if you have year-round asthma there is an allergy to house-dust mites, and if it happens in the spring or summer the allergen is pollen. As Professor Jonathan Brostoff, a leading international authority on allergies, has pointed out, it is scandalous that 90 per cent of children in Britain with asthma are known to have allergies and yet only a tiny minority of them will ever have a skin-prick test.

Factors in the home which may increase asthmatic symptoms:

- Cooking with gas
- Air fresheners
- Fly sprays
- Toilet cleaner
- Fresh paint

Treatments

Drugs that treat asthma provoke a great deal of controversy and there are campaigners who argue passionately against them. There is also an argument put forward by the alternative medicines' lobby which suggests that the drugs are dangerous. Obviously, it's up to everyone to make up their own mind about such treatments, but the truth is that there is now a substantial amount of scientific evidence to back the use of such drugs.

Any medication has the possibility of side effects and not every drug will work for everyone, but looking at the large-scale trials that have been done, it is clear that, for the most part, they do work – and are vastly better than what was available to sufferers twenty or thirty years ago. There are men and women now in their fifties who remember having to miss many months of school because their asthma was so bad they were permanently short of breath, to the point of being disabled by the condition. The former British Prime Minister John Major lost his mother to a violent asthma attack, after several spells in hospital, because her condition could not be kept under control.

However, in the treatment of asthma, medication is only part of the story. What is also becoming clear is that health services across the world could do more to offer different kinds of relief. Breathing exercises work for many people, yet are rarely taught by doctors (see Buteyko Method, page 161). Making simple changes to the home so that it contains fewer allergens and is more conducive to good health would be achievable for most people, but is never properly discussed within a doctor's surgery.

A revolution in medication began in the 1960s, when anti-inflammatory drugs began to appear. Scientists understood that the underlying inflammation of the airways, caused by sensitisation to dust and other substances, was causing the majority of symptoms.

Today, medicinal treatment of asthma can be broken down into two main categories of relievers and preventers. These come in a variety of devices called inhalers, which enable you to breathe the medicine in through your mouth, directly into your lungs.

• Relief treatment

The most common form of relief treatment is through bronchodilators. These work by relaxing the muscles in the walls of the airways, which allows the airways to open. Patients will need these either during an asthma attack, or when their peak flow readings are low, to relieve symptoms, and before exercise to reduce the risk of an attack.

For some, an asthma spacer can be used in conjunction with their prescribed inhaler. A spacer is a plastic container, usually in two halves that click together. At one end there is a mouthpiece and at the other a hole for the inhaler to fit into. It makes the inhaler easier to use. You don't have to worry about pressing the inhaler and breathing at the same time, which can be tricky for children, and you get more of the measured dose of the medicine since it cannot escape into the air because it is trapped inside the spacer.

A nebuliser, which provides a larger, continuous dose, can also be used. Nebulisers work by vaporising a dose of medication in a saline solution into a steady stream of foggy vapour, which the patient inhales continuously until the full dosage is administered.

Nebulisers may be helpful to some patients experiencing a severe attack. Such patients may not be able to inhale deeply, so regular inhalers may not be able to deliver medication deeply into the lungs, even on repeated attempts. Since a nebuliser delivers the medication continuously, it is thought that the first few inhalations may relax the airways enough to allow the following inhalations to draw in more medication.

Bronchodilators

These come in the form of both short-acting and long-acting relievers. The short-acting Beta-agonists work for between two to six hours, and the one most commonly prescribed is Ventolin, also known as salbutamol. Doctors increasingly feel that these should be used only when they are needed, not on a regular, routine basis, because if someone is using their inhaler as a 'quick fix' it means that the underlying problem is not being controlled and they probably need to go onto a preventer as well.

One of the major side effects of this type of medication has been tremors, although this problem has been greatly reduced due to the inhaled delivery which allows the drugs to target the lungs directly. Another side effect can be the risk of heart problems, such as an elevated heart rate or blood pressure, due to the way the drugs work. However, thanks to recent advances, these side effects have become less common. The crucial lesson for patients to learn is that these type of medicines should not be used all the time, because otherwise their effectiveness in relieving symptoms can actually decline.

The other form of bronchodilators which are becoming increasingly more common are the long-acting relievers, all of which are inhaled. These include oxitropium, salmeterol and eformoterol. These have made a big difference in many people's treatments, and are now being offered within combination medicines to alleviate symptoms.

Short- versus long-acting relievers?

Debate has been raging about the safety of long-acting relievers or LABAs – long-acting Beta-agonists. These drugs can give patients much better cover from the symptoms during the day and night. They were developed twenty years ago as a rescue remedy for patients with severe asthma and work by opening the airways for up to twelve hours and preventing symptoms when the usual treatments fail to work.

However, there have been concerns that long-acting relievers may actually end up exacerbating the underlying inflammation. In July 2006, the US Food and Drug Administration put out a 'black-box' warning on the drugs, saying that in certain cases they could actually cause severe attacks and death – but many experts felt the warning was unfair because it was based on cases where some of the patients were not on regular prevention medication and were therefore inherently more at risk in the first place.

A review carried out by the Cochrane Collaboration in the UK in 2007 looked at the current information available from trials and studies and concluded that: 'regular use of long-acting Beta-agonist bronchodilator agents in patients with chronic asthma on regular preventer medication gives better control of asthma than regular use of short-acting Beta-agonist bronchodilator agents.'

However, there remain concerns about children using LABAs because some scientists believe that their regular use may be affecting the underlying condition. In January 2007, the British medicines safety watchdog began their own investigation into these widely prescribed asthma drugs, because of reservations about their safety record.

The Medicines and Healthcare Products Regulatory Agency will review the benefits and risks of long-acting Beta-agonists and, crucially, the panel will also consider whether genetic factors may play a part in how well, or badly, patients respond to the drugs. There is a view that the drugs may actually exacerbate breathing problems in some sufferers.

Around 1.4 million people in Britain are thought to be on LABAs and, generally speaking, GPs see the medications as an important treatment for controlling the condition which affects four million adults and one million children in Britain alone.

> Experts were drawn to the attention of a large US study of more than 26,000 patients carried out by one of the LABA manufacturers, GlaxoSmithKline. The Salmeterol Multicentre Asthma Research Trial began in 1996 and trials were stopped in 2003 after early analysis showed more respiratory-related deaths among those on the drug salmeterol than other asthma medication. When the US Food and Drug Administration issued the 'black-box' health warning, they said that even though LABAs decrease the frequency of asthma episodes, the medicines may make asthma episodes more severe when they occur. In Britain, unlike the U.S., most patients are on the safer form of the drug, which is the combination inhaler of salmeterol or another LABA, formoterol, with a steroid, which help reduce inflammation, so that symptoms, such as wheezing, are more likely to be well controlled.

However, there are concerns that a large subset of asthma sufferers may carry a gene variant which makes them particularly unsuitable for the drugs. Experts in Scotland studied 546 young people who were attending asthma clinics around Tayside. They found that one in seven cases had a particular genotype which predisposed them to an exacerbated condition. One of the scientists involved, respiratory physician Professor Brian Lipworth, said: 'I feel it is time to reappraise what we are doing with these drugs. For a lot of patients, LABAs in a combination inhaler are very good news. I prescribe them myself, but only to those who really need them. I think there are potential problems.' He also added that there was very little evidence to support using the drugs for children.

Pharmaceutical giant GlaxoSmithKline is adamant that the drugs have a very good safety record. Darrell Baker, head of the company's respiratory medicine development centre, said it was about to begin a trial looking at salmeterol to investigate whether there are specific genes that make some patients more vulnerable to the drugs.

He said: 'It is a question that we hope to answer and that is why we have a very major study under way. At the moment, the data from other studies is very conflicting, and the data we have looked at doesn't suggest there is this difference in response to salmeterol, but we do need to look at it.'

Theophylline-type drugs

Patients who are using a steroid inhaler but are still having symptoms may be given theophylline to help them breathe more easily. Theophylline is a drug that helps your airways open up so you can breathe more easily in the morning and evening. It's long-acting and works by relaxing the muscles in your airways. You can take theophylline as a pill or as syrup. It can also be injected.

Emergency relief

A form of emergency relief is an inhaler containing adrenaline or epinephrine. These are used for patients who have a severe form of asthma and may suffer a serious allergic reaction. When used solely as a relief medication, inhaled epinephrine has been shown to work against an attack. In the USA, some of these medications can be bought over the counter, without a prescription.

There are also anti-cholinergic medications, such as ipratropium bromide, which may be used instead. They have no cardiac side effects and so can be used in patients with a history of heart problems, however, they take up to an hour to achieve their full effect and are not as powerful as the LABAs. They have a mixed reliever and preventer effect.

• Prevention medication

The great advance for many patients has been the ability to keep the inflammation, and therefore the symptoms, at bay by using a prevention medication such as an inhaled corticosteroid, a form of steroid. Many people are anxious about taking a steroid, but the type used to help ease the symptoms of asthma are completely different from the anabolic steroids used by bodybuilders – and there is little doubt that they are effective.

Corticosteroids work by reducing the swelling of the lining of the airways and are prescribed to anyone who has frequent (greater than twice a week) need of relievers or who has severe symptoms. Most countries now have guidelines which state that prevention drugs must be given to keep symptoms controlled in all asthma patients, and that this is the best way of preventing the complications that can occur. The difficulty is that when you feel fine, it is hard to see the point of taking a medicine. However, with these drugs, it's important to keep using the prevention medication even when you're well, for long-term improvement.

The preventers usually come in brown inhalers, to distinguish them from the relief inhalers which are usually blue. Inhaled glucocorticoids are the most widely used of the prevention medications and normally come as inhaler devices (ciclesonide, beclomethasone, budesonide, flunisolide, fluticasone, mometasone and triamcinolone).

The possible side effects of long-term use of corticosteroids include a redistribution of fat, increased appetite, possible blood glucose problems and weight gain. In particular, high doses of steroids may cause osteoporosis. As a result, inhaled steroids are generally used for prevention, as their smaller doses are targeted to reach the lungs unlike the higher doses of oral preparations. Nevertheless, patients on high doses of inhaled steroids may still require prophylactic (preventative) treatment to prevent osteoporosis.

Leukotriene modifiers

These are the newest class of drugs for the treatment of asthma. Leukotrienes are chemical compounds that contribute to airway obstruction and they are released during the inflammatory process (see Chapter One, pages 19–20). These drugs block the body's production of leukotrienes and so prevent inflammation and help keep airways open. Drugs in this class include:

- montelukast (brand name Singulair)
- zafirlukast (Accolate)
- zileuton (Zyflo)

Unfortunately, there are no clinical trials which directly compare these three drugs in asthma patients, but all three medications have been shown to be effective in the treatment of asthma. The one which your doctor prescribes will depend on your age, the severity of the asthma and other medical conditions. The most recent asthma guidelines from the U.S. – the National Asthma Education and Prevention Program – states that leukotriene modifiers are an alternative option for patients with mild, persistent asthma, and can also be used in combination with low- to medium-dose inhaled corticosteroids for those with moderate, persistent asthma.

Cromoglycate drugs

These are compounds that are used against several allergies including hayfever.

For asthmatics, the drug is given in the form of an inhaler, and works by preventing the release of some chemicals from the mast cells, a type of cell that is found throughout the body as well as in the lungs, nose and eyelids. In general, it has few side effects, but these can include throat irritation and coughing. Taking a Beta-adrenergic bronchodilator (see page 81) five minutes before using cromoglycate can prevent these side effects.

 Watch out for aspirin

Some 10 per cent of asthmatics are badly affected by aspirin. For most people, aspirin is perfectly safe, but anyone with asthma needs to be aware of the potential danger. The signs that you are having a bad reaction to the drug include: a feeling of exhaustion, sickness or diarrhoea, tightness in the chest, red eyes or flushing. You may not experience all of these symptoms, which can take between thirty minutes to two hours to develop. If you, or a member of your family with asthma, experience any of these reactions after taking aspirin, ring immediately for an ambulance. If you have an adrenaline inhaler, you should use this too.

Asthma at work

Every year in the UK, up to 3,000 people develop asthma because they are exposed to dangerous substances at work. This is called occupational asthma.

Approximately 750,000 people with asthma find that exposure to chemicals at work makes their asthma worse.

Chemicals called isocyanates are the most common cause of occupational asthma in the UK. There are many jobs in which you might be exposed to isocyanates, particularly spray painting, foam moulding using adhesives, and making foundry cores and surface coatings.

Below is a list of the substances that can exacerbate the condition:

- Dust from flour and grain. Industrial baking, farm work and grain transport.

- Wood dust, particularly from hardwood and western red cedar. Carpentry, joinery and sawmilling.

- Colophony – this is widely present in soldering fumes, but also in glues and home floor cleaners. Electronics industry.

- Dust from latex rubber. Any job involving latex gloves, such as nursing or dentistry.

- Dust from insects and animals, and from products containing them. Laboratory work, farm work or work with shellfish.

Children's asthma

Although several medications are available to help children maintain asthma control, clinical trials directly comparing them have not been conducted. In fact, current recommendations in national and international asthma guidelines are based either on studies of single treatments compared to a placebo in children or on comparison studies in adults.

However, in 2006, researchers compared for the first time the effectiveness and safety of three different asthma medicines for initial daily therapy for school-aged children with mild to moderate persistent asthma. These were a low-dose inhaled corticosteroid (200 mcg fluticasone a day); a combination of a lower dose inhaled corticosteroid and an inhaled long-acting Beta-agonist (100 mcg fluticasone each morning plus 50mcg salmeterol twice daily), and a leukotriene receptor antagonist (montelukast).

Studying 285 children, aged between six and fourteen, researchers at the Childhood Asthma Research and Education Network of the National Heart,

Lung, and Blood Institute (NHLBI) in Bethesda, USA, found that after forty-eight weeks, inhaled corticosteroids were the most effective initial daily therapy for children with mild to moderate persistent asthma. They also found no significant adverse growth effects among any of the medicines studied.

For children, it is also very important to learn how to deal with the different problems that can come with an asthma attack. If they panic, it can make the situation much worse so both the parents and the child must learn how to respond in the right way. Relaxation techniques such as meditation and yoga can help with this (see pages 157–162). Exercise is also important because if the child is inactive, spending their days in front of the TV, the lungs are not exercised, and they can put on weight, which aggravates the condition. If the asthma is induced by exercise, they can use their relief medication prior to any activity to help overcome this.

 Swimming pools

A number of parents I have spoken to think that their children's condition becomes worse when they go to certain indoor swimming pools. This is partly backed up by research suggesting that there may be an increase in symptoms.

A study carried out in Belgium looked at teenagers from twenty-one countries across Europe, and found the greater the number of indoor pools, the higher the rates of childhood asthma and wheeze. The rates rose by around 2–3 per cent for every indoor chlorinated swimming pool per 100,000 people. The researchers believe the key could be exposure to chlorine, which is used to keep pools clean. They also say the long-term effects of chlorine by-products on children's respiratory health should be thoroughly evaluated and that pools should be properly ventilated and levels of chlorine by-products regulated. There is also some evidence that chlorine in pools can react with sweat or urine to create harmful fumes which can damage lungs.

The study also found that children who regularly attend indoor pools accumulate proteins that in high quantities can cause damage to cells in the lungs.

The challenge of teenagers

The point about adolescence is that you feel you're invincible and that the rules that apply to others don't really apply to you. The problem is that not following those rules, when it comes to asthma, can leave you feeling much worse and sometimes in danger.

Quite often the symptoms of asthma will change as children enter puberty and experience the usual rushes of hormones and emotions. Males in late adolescence and early adulthood tend to find their symptoms actually become less obvious. Girls, however, may find that their symptoms alter according to the time of the month as their hormones change. The overriding problem, however, is that teenagers often don't tell their parents or doctor about any symptoms they may have. In fact, their lives are so full of homework demands and social pressures, and their priorities are so different, that they may not recognise themselves when they are beginning to fall ill.

Nancy Ostrom, an associate clinical professor of paediatrics at the University of California, USA, believes that the trick lies in recognising the subtle clues that the condition is not being kept under control. 'That is the challenge, really,' she says. 'If you are hearing them cough a lot at night, if they seem very sleepy the next morning, if they seem to have had a lot of colds lasting longer than usual, or if they are finding exercise hard – all these could be important signs that the condition is not being controlled adequately.' She also makes the point that teenagers often won't admit to their parents that they are not taking their medication regularly.

Nancy Ostrom's key aim is to persuade teenagers themselves to look out for the signs. 'Adolescents often don't tell me what is going on. Also, they may not realise themselves that when they've been trying to catch a Frisbee with their friends, and they can't run that fast or that far, that it may be their asthma. So I tell them that a lot of the American Youth Olympics swimming team actually has exercise-induced asthma, and they manage it to the point where they are able to be elite athletes. I don't expect my patients to become Olympic qualifiers, but I also don't expect their asthma to become an excuse for not leading a full, active and fun life.'

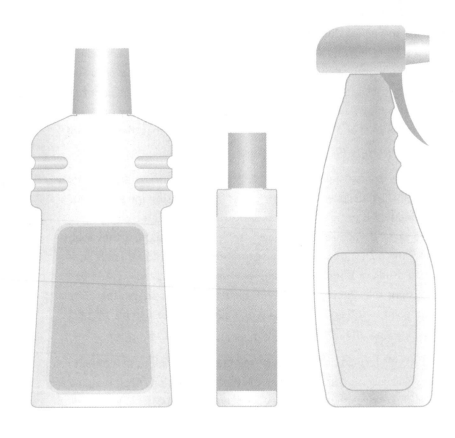

CHAPTER SIX
MULTIPLE CHEMICAL SENSITIVITY

Of all the allergic conditions that cause controversy, multiple chemical sensitivity (MCS) is the one which arouses the most passion. There are a growing number of people who believe they react very badly to a whole range of common substances that we come into contact with in our daily lives. The fumes from a petrol exhaust, the smell of nail varnish or a tabletop cleaned with disinfectant are substances which sufferers say can cause a range of symptoms from tiredness, headaches and dizzy spells through to aching joints, chest pain and digestive problems.

Some people with MCS say that they were injured by a single exposure to chemicals. Others say that they developed an intolerance to chemicals over time. But the symptoms can include migraine headaches, itchy eyes and throat, nausea, muscle aches, anxiety and insomnia.

Jenny, 42, from Sussex, UK, starts to feel ill as soon as she steps outside. 'I do believe it is the fumes coming from the car and lorry exhausts,' she explains. 'After an hour or so, I start to get a throbbing head, and sometimes a dizziness comes over me.

'When I visit my parents in the countryside, there is never a problem. It's only when I'm commuting into work, walking to the rail station and then taking a bus ride, that I get these symptoms. I've talked to my GP who is quite sympathetic, but was told there is nothing that can be done. Avoiding traffic pollution would only be possible if I could work from home and, as

I'm an office manager, that really isn't an option. I'm quite worried that the symptoms may get worse.'

Some believe MCS simply doesn't exist, with many doctors and scientists saying it is a psychosomatic illness, meaning one which has physical characteristics caused largely by psychological factors. They say it is described by patients who put down a range of illnesses to numerous chemical exposures because they cannot get any other kind of diagnosis.

Unlike food intolerance, where there are proper studies and trials, there is no scientific proof of a link between these chemicals and particular conditions. This is partly because it isn't an easy area to investigate, but also because the symptoms are difficult to define since they include confusion, dizziness and headaches.

Over the years, the phenomenon has been given various labels, such as universal allergy, 20th-century syndrome, and total allergy syndrome, and recently a group of experts meeting at the World Health Organisation suggested a new name – idiopathic environmental intolerances. They decided that the term MCS 'makes an unsupported judgement on the causation' and does not refer to a 'clinically defined disease'.

Proponents of the case for MCS would point to two recent studies which have tried to address the issue. In Tokyo, Dr Mariko Saito and her colleagues at the Department of Psychosomatic Medicine at the University looked at how 'real' the condition was. They compared eighteen patients with MCS and twelve healthy controls (people who were unaffected) and measured their responses over one week when exposed to various chemicals. They looked at how they reacted to both physical and psychological symptoms. They concluded that 'MCS patients do not have either somatic (bodily) or psychologic symptoms under chemical-free conditions and symptoms may be provoked only when exposed to chemicals'.

In another study, carried out in Canada in 2004, researchers looked at 203 women, all MCS sufferers, and 162 controls. They found that blood tests revealed that genetic differences relating to the body's detoxification processes were present more often in those with MCS than those without. People with two specific genes (CYP2D6 and NAT2) were eighteen times more likely to have MCS than those without the genes. The authors concluded that 'a genetic predisposition for MCS may involve altered biotransformation of environmental chemicals'.

Substances often blamed for causing MCS include:
- Aerosols
- Tobacco smoke
- Petrol and oil fumes
- Nail varnish
- Plastic content in clingfilm
- Air-fresheners
- Disinfectant
- Household polish
- Newspaper print
- Pesticides
- Aftershave and perfume

93

Is there an answer?

None of this controversy does much to help patients who believe that they are sensitive to particular chemicals, so what should they do if they are in this situation?

There is only one real solution and that is to avoid the chemicals as much as possible. There is no diagnostic test, such as a skin-prick test, they can undergo, so it really is trial and error.

Some chemicals will be much easier to avoid than others. As so many countries are now introducing bans on smoking in public places, it will be easier for people to avoid cigarette smoke, for example. If you think you might be sensitive to the usual detergents and cleaning materials in the home, remove them for a couple of weeks and resort to water and an unscented, detergent-free washing-up liquid to see if your symptoms subside.

Chemicals are all around us, they are essential for many goods and there is a limit to what you can do to avoid exposure. But if you suspect that it may be formaldehyde causing your problems, you should stay away from all paper, photographs, antiperspirants and a range of other goods. Formaldehyde is also contained in many building materials such as insulation and, therefore, is very difficult to avoid.

Perhaps the best advice is to try and avoid the chemicals as much as possible but not to become too stressed about what can't be avoided. Eat well, exercise as much as you can and try to keep it in perspective, rather than seeing the world around you as 'the enemy'.

 Theron Randolph, father of clinical ecology

The term 'chemical sensitivities' was first coined by the pioneering allergist Theron Randolph, a Chicago-based doctor who went against the theories of the day to advance research into how the body would be affected by different chemicals.

During a series of studies with patients, he saw that exposure to low levels of modern synthetic chemicals caused a wide range of symptoms. His observations were controversial because he challenged the idea that a group of people would all have the same response to particular doses of chemicals.

Dr Randolph's technique was to interview his patients thoroughly. He asked many questions and kept his face expressionless, regardless of their answers, while typing their responses on a manual typewriter.

But much of the questioning was also about foods people ate daily or even repeatedly throughout the day, as well as possible toxic exposures in the home and at work. What he was most worried about was the kind of chemicals that people were exposed to frequently.

To unmask the allergy, Dr Randolph guessed the suspected allergens, based on the results of his interview. He then strictly isolated his client from these suspected allergens for a period of time – usually five days. During this period, the allergen had the opportunity to be detoxified from the body. Next, Dr Randolph had the client return to his office to eat the suspected foods, inhale the suspicious chemicals, and so on. The results were dramatic. With the allergy unmasked, the response was often acute.

He won acclaim for his seminal book, *Human Ecology and Susceptibility to the Chemical Environment* in 1962, two years before the American environmentalist Rachel Carson published *Silent Spring*. But he was also heavily criticised for his methods and theories. What is not in doubt is that he was a pioneer in environmental medicine and was correctly questioning the effect of so many chemicals on our health at a time when people were being told very little about the downside of industrialisation.

CHAPTER SEVEN
ECZEMA

Eczema is the name given to a group of skin conditions that can affect people of all ages. It's extremely common, and is becoming even more so, along with the rise in other allergic conditions. In the United Kingdom, up to one fifth of all children of school age have eczema, along with about one in twelve of the adult population.

The condition is characterised by an itchy rash and by blisters that dry out and become scaly. The skin itself becomes very dry and itchy, causing a great deal of pain and discomfort – this itchiness can be almost unbearable at times. The most common form of eczema is known as atopic dermatitis, which is different from contact dermatitis (see pages 107–113).

Constant scratching can also cause the skin to split, leaving it prone to infection. In infected eczema, the skin may crack and weep. For young children, in particular, the condition can be profoundly distressing not only for the physical discomfort it causes but also because it may make them stand out from other children and can mean having to wear bandages. For parents trying to deal with it, this skin condition can be exhausting. British TV presenter Fiona Phillips has talked about her experiences in dealing with her son Mackenzie's chronic eczema: 'For a while I seemed to live under a cloud of despair and my perspective was blurred through sheer exhaustion,' she says. 'I just couldn't see an end to our chaotic life with eczema. From the planning involved in simple trips out with packing creams, bandages, scissors and special foods, to the simple but stressful things like not being able to cuddle Mackenzie because he was so sore. It became overwhelming at times.'

Fiona, who is a patron of the National Eczema Society in the UK, hopes to raise awareness of the condition which can have a huge impact on families but is still little understood. Children can often wake several times a night because they have scratched so much and need more cream to be applied. This can take its toll on the whole household and the amount of attention needed to be given to the child with the eczema can result in other siblings feeling left out.

What happens with eczema?

98

For reasons that are not fully understood, the skin becomes dry because too much moisture is lost from its upper layer. This means that the skin has no protection and any foreign organism, such as bacteria, can invade and cause inflammation. Sufferers go through periods when symptoms flare up and are severe and times when there are no symptoms at all (known as remission).

However, the exact nature of this allergy is a bit of a puzzle. Most people with the condition have raised levels of the antibody IgE, as a blood test would reveal, and which would also be demonstrated by suffering reactions to common allergens when given a skin-prick test. However, when more intensive tests are done, it often turns out that patients are not actually allergic to a specific substance. This has made some doctors question whether eczema really is a truly allergic condition, or perhaps some other problem within the immune system.

House-dust mites, cats and dogs, and cow's milk are common allergens for an an eczema sufferer, often resulting in a rash. But food intolerances are also common, although there may be a delay of several hours between ingesting the food and the rash appearing.

What is undeniable is that the condition is on the increase. More than 15 million people in the United States have eczema. Many of them will also have another allergy such as asthma or hayfever, and possibly also a food intolerance.

Symptoms of eczema occur repeatedly. The most common signs are:
- Dry, extremely itchy skin
- Blisters with oozing and crusting
- Redness of the skin around the blisters
- Raw areas of the skin from scratching, which may even lead to bleeding
- Dry, leathery areas with more or less pigment than their normal skin tone (called lichenification)

Eczema in children under two years old generally begins on the cheeks, elbows or knees. In adults, it tends to be located on the inside surfaces of the knees and elbows.

The cause of eczema is thought to be a combination of hereditary (genetic) and environmental factors. This means that factors such as allergies can cause eczema in susceptible people. It is also known that eczema is linked to hayfever and asthma (see Chapters Four and Five). Exposure to certain irritants and allergens in the environment can worsen symptoms, as can dryness of the skin, exposure to water, temperature changes and stress.

Around two-thirds of cases happen before the age of one, and around 90 per cent by the age of five, but it can also appear in adulthood. There are some risk factors that have been identified which include living in a climate with low humidity and having a family history of allergies to plants, chemicals or food.

Treatment

The goals when treating eczema are to heal the skin, to reduce symptoms, prevent skin damage and stop it flaring up. The treatment pathway varies depending on the patient's age, symptoms and also their general health. Following a set routine to try and restore the proper protective layer of the skin and avoid it getting worse is absolutely essential. If you use complementary remedies, your main goal should be to calm down the inflammation and control the symptoms.

• Steroid creams

These creams and ointments have different degrees of strength, from mild to very potent. Known correctly as corticosteroids, these drugs are successful at delivering the treatment to exactly where it is needed but they do need to be used correctly. Some parents feel as if they are walking a tightrope at times: too much cream and you may have a side effect, such as an outbreak of spots or, in the long term thinning of the skin, and too little and it won't control the underlying problem.

Take the doctor's advice and use the kind of cream that is necessary for you or your child. Some patients will only need a mild one, or an over-the-counter lotion which can heal up the dry and scaly lesions. Others may need a much more potent treatment to control severe eczema. Patients and their families have become fearful of steroids, worried about their possible side effects, but if they are used properly they do work. The creams are known as 'topical medication' as they are applied to the skin. They don't tackle the allergy itself, but instead deal with the inflammation by calming down the immune response.

Chronic, thickened areas of skin may be treated with ointments or creams that contain tar compounds, as well as corticosteroids (medium to very high potency) and ingredients that lubricate or soften the skin.

Short courses of steroid tablets may also be prescribed to reduce inflammation in some severe cases. In very rare instances, medications that suppress the immune system (called immunosuppressants such as cyclosporine) may be considered in adults with extremely severe eczema who do not respond to oral steroids. Antihistamines may also be recommended for use at night to prevent night-time scratching. These medications may cause drowsiness.

The good news is that a new class of skin medications have come along, known as topical immunomodulators (TIMs). These medications are steroid-free. The most common are tacrolimus, for severe to moderate eczema, and pimecrolimus, for milder forms, suitable for children. Studies have shown as high as an 80 per cent success rate using these new medications. It gives doctors another kind of treatment to try if patients are not getting on well with steroid creams, but they cost a great deal more and so tend to be prescribed as a second-line treatment.

Mind over matter?

It's known that gaining some control over levels of stress and anxiety, as well as treating depression, can prevent eczema flaring up. A new form of psychological therapy, known as cognitive behavioural therapy (CBT) has been shown to help. However, just being aware of the dangers of stress can help you to avoid those situations. When you become upset or angry, the blood vessels close to the skin dilate, and that can bring on itching. This is not to say that eczema is 'all in the mind', just that psychological factors can have quite an impact on the intensity of the symptoms.

Avoidance measures

Anything that aggravates the symptoms should be avoided. This includes allergens such as pollen, house-dust mites and animal fur (especially dog and cat hair) and irritants to the skin – the most common being wool, synthetic fibres, soaps and detergents, perfumes, cosmetics, lanolin, certain chemicals such as chlorine and solvents (including mineral oil), cigarette smoke, dust and sand. Try to keep the home environment cool, with stable temperature and humidity.

101

Remember to:

- Avoid hot baths or showers as this can exacerbate the skin.
- Wash or bathe as quickly as possible to lessen water contact which has a drying effect on the skin.
- Use a mild soap.
- Moisturise. After bathing, it is important to trap the moisture in the skin by applying lubricating cream on the skin while it is damp. Individuals prefer different products. Ointments are greasy and can be difficult to use because they leave marks on clothes, bedding and carpets. They can also make you feel very hot, but some people quite like the greasiness. Others prefer water-based creams. They tend to be white and are more easily used as they can soak into the skin after application. They can be more soothing because they feel cool on the skin and some people find it soothes the itchiness quite quickly.
- In severe cases, moisturiser can also be smeared onto bandages which are then wound around the affected areas at night, to quell the desire to itch, or you can use ready-made 'wet wraps' – ask your doctor for details.
- Keep your child's nails short so that they cannot harm the skin when they are itching.
- If using steroid creams, don't stop them too soon. The skin on the top may look fine but it may be still healing below.
- See a doctor regularly, especially if you are using a strong steroid cream.

Diet

Some patients do feel that their diet has a role to play in affecting symptoms. This is very specific to every individual and should be discussed with your healthcare provider. A doctor, dietician or naturopath, for example, can help you make the necessary dietary changes and determine if the lack of these foods in your diet is reducing the incidence and severity of your eczema.

Some studies have shown that children who are exclusively breastfed for at least four months are less likely to get eczema. Recent studies suggest that babies whose mothers used probiotics during pregnancy and while breastfeeding were less likely to have eczema up to two years of age.

102

Paying attention to what you or your child eat and the effect it has on the skin may help you pinpoint your own particular triggers. Foods that are said to provoke flare-ups include peanuts, milk, soy, fish and eggs. Fried foods and hydrogenated oils may not help – on the other hand, fresh fruits and vegetables, wholegrains, and foods rich in Omega 3 fatty acids (such as nuts, flax, seeds, and cold-water fish) may reduce inflammation in those without sensitivities to these foods.

Supplements to consider and discuss with your doctor include gamma-linolenic acid, or GLA, which is an Omega-6 essential fatty acid. Studies are mixed but there is some evidence that the metabolism of essential fatty acids is abnormal in people with eczema, resulting in low levels of GLA. Several early studies suggested that GLA, derived from evening primrose oil (EPO), is beneficial for relieving symptoms associated with this skin condition such as itching, redness and scaling. However, more recent studies have not had the same positive results. Whether or not GLA or EPO supplements work for eczema may be very individual. Talk to your dermatology nurse or doctor to decide if it is safe and worthwhile for you to try this for your eczema.

The situation in Australia

You might think that being in a hot and sunny climate with lots of fresh air would leave a society far less prone to the condition, but there are at least 1 million adult Australians suffering from atopic eczema. And there is definitely a price to be paid. Some research carried out in 2002 showed that adult patients spent an average out-of-pocket amount of $425 per year on products, as well as an average of $121 a year on medical consultations. Also, 40 per cent of the eighty-five adults who were monitored for a year were using four or more products to treat their eczema. According to Heather Jacobs, President of the Eczema Association of Australia: 'This common, frustrating and often debilitating skin disease can have a significant physical and emotional toll on sufferers and their carers' quality of life, while also proving costly to the public purse.'

The vast majority of sufferers put stressful situations as the reason for flare-ups of the condition. Lead study investigator and dermatologist, Professor Robin Marks, from St Vincent's Hospital in Melbourne says: 'Of the sixty-six responses from participants who said that a life event had made their atopic eczema worse, 64 per cent cited increased stress as a reason. The weather, hormones, treatments, holidays and illness were other reasons voiced by participants for the deterioration of their skin condition.' For 21 per cent of those taking part in the study, their eczema was a source of embarrassment or made them feel self conscious.

 Felice's story

Felice Oxborrow has found a way of helping her son overcome much of his eczema, thanks to both conventional medicine and complementary herbal remedies and food supplements. She trained as a scientist and was initially highly sceptical of any kind of complementary medicine but has been won over by the fact that, for her ten-year-old boy Matthew, the treatments seem to work.

'The first thing I noticed about him as a baby was that once a month, he would be physically sick. It was as if something was accumulating inside him which needed to come out. Then, as a toddler, he began to suffer from asthma, not severely, but enough to worry me. He was put on a nebuliser [see page 81] and that helped a lot. But it was the eczema that troubled him most. It appeared mostly on his knees and on his elbows. It was never so severe that we had to wet-wrap him and he was never hospitalised with it but it did affect him.'

For five years, Felice and her husband Mike used the emollient and steroid creams to rub into the raised red areas, but it didn't seem to be getting any better. A friend then suggested a naturopath, who worked in their home town of Richmond, Surrey, and Matthew went along to have sensitivity tests. The naturopath suggested that Matthew was reacting badly to some of the major food groups and should stay away from yeast, milk, cheese, sugar and chocolate.

'At first it seemed like a really major undertaking, particularly cutting out sugar which was a bit of nightmare but we decided that the whole family would follow the same diet,' recalled Felice. As well as switching to soya and eating many different foods, the naturopath also gave her a herbal mixture for Matthew to have once a day and supplements containing the essential fatty acids (Omega 3, 6, and 9) as well as a probiotic – *lactobacillus sporogenes*. 'We noticed that his temperament altered. In the past, he was quite often either very happy or very upset but after the change in diet he became calmer, maybe because of the lack of sugar,' says Felice. 'But we also noticed a big difference in his eczema – it was far more mild.

'These days, at the age of ten he gets just a little on the knees and nothing around the elbows. I don't know which of the different approaches has worked for him – whether it is the change in diet, or the herbs or the multivitamins or a combination of all three – but I'm convinced they help him, even though I don't know how they work exactly.'

A scientific explanation

Scientists moved closer to understanding the causes of eczema and asthma in 2006 after discovering a genetic mutation in the skin of people who have the conditions. Researchers in Scotland discovered that around two-thirds of eczema cases and a quarter of asthma cases carry a genetic mutation that is involved in causing skin to become dry and scaly.

The work of Professor Irwin McLean and Dr Frances Smith in Dundee centred on a gene which produces a protein called fillagrin – normally found in large quantities in the outermost layers of the skin. This protein is essential for good health as it helps to form a protective layer at the surface of the skin that keeps water in and foreign organisms out.

When people have either a reduction or complete absence of this protein, it leads to an impaired formation of the skin barrier. As a result, the skin dries out too easily and the outer layers of the skin are poorly formed and constantly flake off. In people with fillagrin mutations, foreign substances can easily enter the skin and be picked by the immune system, producing a response. For people with an immune system which is primed through their genes to develop 'leaky skin', this would then explain the link with asthma, where foreign substances later enter the lungs.

The work carried out by Professor McLean and his team at Dundee University studied four groups of people: fifty-two Irish children with eczema; 604 Scottish children with asthma; 372 Danish children whose mothers have asthma and fifteen families with a condition called *ichthyosis vulgaris*, which causes flaky and scaly skin. In all groups they found that two different mutations to the fillagrin gene were much more common than in the general population. Their findings were reported in the journal, *Nature Genetics*.

Although around one in ten people of European origin carry one of the mutations, the study found that around two-thirds of the Irish eczema patients had it. However, Professor McLean said that other environmental factors, such as central heating or increased cleanliness, might also play a role as some people with one of the mutations do not develop eczema at all. It is known that around half of eczema patients go on to develop asthma, accounting for about a quarter of asthma cases, and the Dundee study opens up the possibility that a treatment that targets the fillagrin mutation might also be used to treat some forms of asthma.

Margaret Cox, Chief Executive of the UK's National Eczema Society, said: 'To discover that eczema patients don't have the gene which should protect the skin by keeping water in and keeping foreign organisms out is a real step forward. Above all, it answers the age-old question asked by most eczema sufferers, "why?".

'Understanding the genetic basis of skin diseases such as eczema means that in the future, healthcare professionals will be armed with more and better information and we can tackle the cause rather than simply treat the symptoms of a previously 'incurable' skin condition.'

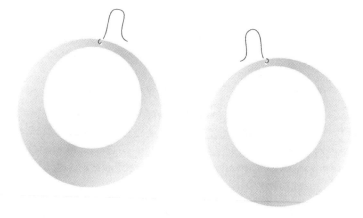

CHAPTER EIGHT
CONTACT DERMATITIS

Contact dermatitis is a condition, primarily a rash, that develops when the body's immune system reacts against a substance that comes in contact with the skin. It usually develops over a period of time where the skin has had repeated contact with the substance.

One very common reaction is to nickel, which is found in earrings, buttons on jeans and many bits of metal that are commonly worn. Or it could be perfume or rubber or hair dye that causes the problem. The most important step is to find out what it is that is causing the rash or the symptoms in the first place.

There are two types of condition: allergic contact dermatitis (ACD), which is the most common kind, and irritant contact dermatitis (ICD).

The most common allergens include:

- Nickel
- Fragrances
- Rubber
- Some plants
- Formaldehyde
- Hair chemicals

An allergic response

In allergic contact dermatitis, the skin reacts to something that has touched it at that site. Unlike most allergic reactions, the trigger is an external one, rather than something that is inhaled or swallowed. This type of skin allergy begins with a process called sensitisation. When the allergen manages to penetrate the outer layer of the skin, it reaches the cells beneath. This process lasts from four days to three weeks, and during this time there are no signs of skin damage.

108

Once penetrated, the allergenic substance combines with natural skin proteins. This is then carried throughout the body setting up an immune reaction. This means that you react to the next exposure. If you seem to react the first time you are exposed to an agent, you probably were exposed before without knowing.

Allergic contact dermatitis usually shows redness, swelling and water blisters, from tiny to large. The blisters may break, forming crusts and scales. Untreated, the skin may darken and become leathery and cracked. This reaction can be difficult to distinguish from other rashes, especially after it has been present for a while.

 case study ──────────────────────────────

> Susan, a 36-year-old British woman now living in the south of France, started to come out in a red rash over her arms when she moved house. She realised that she had changed to a different kind of soap which produced the reaction. 'The problem was that we were painting our new home, so at first I thought it was the paint,' she says. 'I'd never had an allergic reaction in my life before, so it was quite scary.
>
> 'Eventually, I changed to an olive oil soap and that was much better. The rash cleared up but I do notice now that my skin seems to be more sensitive to different perfumes especially if I'm away from home and I use different products.'

────────────────────────────── **case study**

• Nickel

Found in certain metals, nickel is one of the biggest triggers for contact dermatitis and, unfortunately, it is found in a variety of products. Many chrome-plated objects contain enough nickel to produce a reaction in sensitive people. Stainless steel also contains nickel but it is bound in such a way that makes the stainless steel safe for most nickel-sensitive individuals.

For many women, earrings containing nickel can cause earlobe dermatitis, a very common problem. This is the reason why only sterile stainless steel needles should be used for piercing. After your ears have been pierced, you should wear only nickel-free earrings for at least the first three weeks.

Clothing accessories made of nickel such as buckles, zippers, buttons and metal clips can also cause dermatitis. The list of goods to avoid is endless, but at least it is possible to substitute with accessories made from nickel-free materials in most cases.

Sweating increases dermatitis in nickel-sensitive people. In the summer, items containing nickel can cause an itchy, prickly sensation within fifteen to twenty minutes of touching perspiring skin. A rash may appear within a day or two.

• Latex

Latex (rubber) products often cause ACD. For nurses, this is a particular problem because most gloves they have to wear when touching patients are made from rubber. The condition can cause immediate allergic reactions, including itching or burning immediately at the point of contact on the skin. Some people also experience itching and streaming eyes and, occasionally, shortness of breath. This is more common in people who wear tight-fitting rubber gloves, such as medical workers. Rubber gloves may also cause dermatitis on the skin of the hands under the glove. Even leather shoes can cause problems because ingredients in the rubber which are used to hold the shoe together can provoke a reaction. If possible, try to find shoes without rubber in them at all.

Obviously, avoidance of the known allergen is the best policy but if you have to wear protective gloves, opt for vinyl (PVC) ones. If you have no choice but to wear latex gloves, ensure that they are unpowdered and always wear cotton gloves underneath.

• Hair dyes

There has been a lot of controversy in recent years over permanent hair dyes and the chemicals they contain. One of the key ingredients is paraphenylenedeamine (PPDA), currently found in two thirds of hair colourants, which has to be mixed with an oxidizing agent, such as peroxide, before application. Researchers warned in the *British Medical Journal* in 2007 that the chemical can lead to dermatitis on the face and, in severe cases, facial swelling.

People allergic to PPDA really should not use any permanent hair dyes. About one fourth of the people allergic to it are also allergic to ingredients in semi-permanent dyes. If you're not sure about your reaction, always follow the package instructions for a patch test before you use for the first time.

As more and more people dye their hair, the allergic reactions are increasing. Dr John McFadden, a dermatologist at St Thomas' Hospital in London, whose research showed an increase in the condition, said: 'Hair dye allergy may present with mild or severe symptoms. For example, in mild cases there may just be tingling or discomfort of the scalp after hair dyeing. If severe, there may be redness and swelling of the forehead, ears, neck and eyelids; some patients have been hospitalised after an acute attack.'

During the 20th century, allergic reactions to PPDA became such a serious problem that it was banned from hair dyes in Germany, France and Sweden. However, the current European Union legislation allows PPDA to comprise up to 6 per cent of the constituents of hair dyes on the consumer market, as no satisfactory or widely accepted alternatives to these agents are available for use in permanent hair dye.

Market research also confirms that more people are dyeing their hair and are doing so at a younger age. A survey in 1992 by the Japan Soap and Detergent Association found 13 per cent of female high school students, 6 per cent of women in their twenties and 2 per cent of men in their twenties reported using hair colouring products. By 2001, the proportions had increased in these three groups to 41 per cent, 85 per cent, and 33 per cent, respectively.

One alternative for sufferers is to look at organic hair dyes which are now becoming increasingly popular. However, always check the ingredients before you buy to ensure they doesn't contain PPDA.

• Chromates

Compounds containing chromium, called chromates, are commonly responsible for ACD in construction workers and others who have constant contact with cement, leather, some matches, paints and anti-rust compounds. Exposure to chromium is common in jobs in the automobile, welding, foundry, cement, railroad and building repair industries, but sometimes goes unnoticed – or ignored – by employers. However, according to some US statistics, skin disorders comprise more than 45 per cent of all occupationally related diseases. Among all cases of occupational dermatitis, allergic contact dermatitis accounts for about 30 per cent.

111

Irritant Contact Dermatitis

This is not a truly allergic response because it is not an immune reaction, but instead occurs from coming into contact with a substance that directly damages the skin. Sometimes known as 'housewives' eczema', ICD is the most common form of contact dermatitis, causing about 80 per cent of cases, and probably affecting around 1–2 per cent of healthy Europeans. It tends to be caused by physical irritants and particularly affects people who do a lot of work involving chemicals. Mothers of small children, hairdressers, nurses and chefs are very prone to developing this, and the only real solution is to avoid the source of the problem.

What is happening is that certain chemicals, such as detergents, surfactants and some solvents directly prevent the outer layer of the skin, the epidermis, from working properly as a barrier. The chemicals remove the fat emulsion which covers it, causing cellular damage on the underlying areas. They can also increase the water loss within the different layers of the skin, causing them to thin out.

Remember that:

- The longer the substance remains on the skin, the more severe the reaction.
- Many chemicals, including industrial cleaning products and solvents, can cause this condition.
- Household cleaners such as detergents can also cause dermatitis.

Here is a list of different professions and their susceptibility to the substances they come into contact with on a daily basis.

Agriculture workers	Rubber, oats, barley, animal feed, veterinary medications, cement, plants, pesticides, wood preservatives
Artists	Turpentine, pigments, dyes, colophony, epoxy resin
Bartenders	Orange, lemon, lime flavours
Butchers	Nickel, sawdust
Cleaners	Rubber gloves, cleaning products
Construction workers	Chromates, cobalt, rubber and leather gloves, resins, woods
Cooks and caterers	Foods: onions, garlic, spices, flavours, rubber gloves, sodium metabisulphite, lauryl and octyl gallate, formaldehyde
Dry cleaners	Rubber gloves
Electricians	Fluxes, resins, rubber
Florists and gardeners	Plants, pesticides, rubber gloves
Foundry workers	Phenol-and urea-formaldehyde resins, colophony
Hairdressers	Dyes, persulphates, nickel, perfumes, rubber gloves, formaldehyde, resorcinol, pyrogallol
Jewellers	Epoxy resin, metals, soldering fluxes
Mechanics	Rubber gloves, chromates, epoxy resin, antifreeze
Office workers	Rubber, nickel, glue
Photography industry workers	Rubber gloves, colour developers, para-aminophenol, hydroquinone, formaldehyde, sodium metabisulphite, chromates
Printers	Nickel, chromates, cobalt, colophony, formaldehyde, turpentine
Shoemakers	Glues, leather, rubber, turpentine

Treatment

In some countries, it is possible for patients to see a dermatologist, who specialises in skin complaints, but in the UK your first port of call is likely to be your GP. He or she will talk to you about your exposure to different materials, to try and work out the allergen. It is also possible to have a patch test, where a small amount of the suspected chemical or substance is put on your skin to see if you react.

Contact dermatitis usually starts in, and often remains in, the part of your body most in contact with the substance, so the area of affected skin is an important clue to what has caused the rash. If you can't actually avoid exposure to a particular substance, then you should consider either wearing protective clothing or using a barrier cream – although neither of these work as well as complete avoidance.

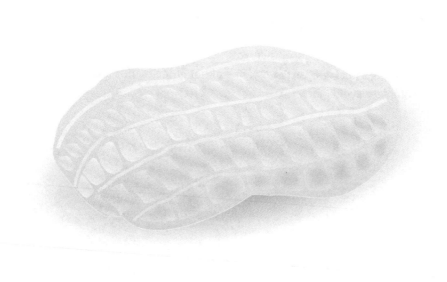

CHAPTER NINE
FOOD ALLERGIES AND INTOLERANCES

❝ **case study** ─────────────────────────────────

Jude, a young teacher living near Sydney, Australia, didn't really understand it when she started to suffer the feelings of a bloated tummy every evening. 'I had always been able to eat absolutely everything – too much in fact. But suddenly I found myself, at the age of 23, with this tummy that felt as tight as a drum and accompanied with terrible cramping pains. The doctor put it down to stress, as my school job was quite demanding at that stage. He suggested taking up yoga or jogging. It was my mother who realised that whenever I had a milky coffee or a cheese sandwich, the pains would follow and in fact they tended to last for at least a day.

'I took myself off dairy products, which wasn't easy as I was addicted to cheese in any form, and I switched to buy soya milk. It has really helped and the pains have disappeared although my stomach still isn't completely right. I saw another doctor, who told me that it is not unusual to develop lactose intolerance in your twenties. For now, I'm going to keep off the dairy. I only wish I had done it earlier and hadn't gone through nearly two years of pretty painful cramps.'

───────────────────────────────── **case study** ❞

Jude is certainly not alone in her experiences. When it comes to the body's reaction to food, there is an enormous amount of confusion surrounding the role diet can play. It seems sad to me that the whole issue of food allergy and intolerance is cloaked in misunderstandings and conflicting arguments. There is enormous medical scepticism about whether intolerances really exist. This is partly a result of the paucity of good scientific studies to prove or disprove the links between food and symptoms.

To those working in the field of allergies, it has become quite clear that many people who live with painful and debilitating symptoms that can't be given an easy diagnosis may indeed be experiencing some kind of reaction to food. But very often it takes years for patients to be helped, often because their condition is put down to depression or stress. In other words, they are told their problem has a psychological origin when, in fact, no one has bothered to investigate whether they may be experiencing a real problem with a particular food which they've eaten every day of their life.

Allergy or intolerance?

Firstly, it is important to clear up the differences between an allergy and an intolerance. A lot of people use the terms interchangeably, but they really are two different conditions. A food allergy is where you have an acute reaction involving the immune system to even a small quantity of a particular food. A few flakes of fish can be enough to make some people very ill indeed. It involves the usual culprit, the antibody IgE (see Chapter One, page 18) which is produced in relation to a foodstuff that is usually harmless. A genuine food allergy is much more rare than an intolerance and tends to be far more serious.

An intolerance to a food appears to build up over time and, essentially, this is a condition in which the immune system does not seem to play a part. It may start in childhood but, as the above case shows, it is also common for adults to find themselves suddenly unable to take in a particular food group. Intolerance does not involve the production of IgE antibodies but is the body's response to a common food, or group of foods, which produces a set of chronic symptoms. These symptoms can be alleviated – or eliminated altogether – simply by cutting out the particular food group in question. It can also be described as idiopathic food intolerance, which means food intolerance with no established mechanism (e.g. no exact cause) but you should be aware of the fact that many doctors dispute its existence.

There is also a condition known as food aversion. This is when people develop an intense dislike, or aversion, to a particular food, for emotional or psychological reasons. The food itself is not producing the symptoms – it is about the associations made by the sufferer with a particular food that causes the problem.

Food allergies

There are very few people who suffer from genuine food allergies, as described above, where the immune system goes into overdrive to fight off particular substances. The one that is most commonly talked about is peanut allergy, which can be life-threatening. However, there are also people who are allergic to rice, which is far more common in Asia than in Europe, and there a number of other foods including fish or shellfish and sesame seeds which provoke severe reactions.

• Nut allergy

Over the past two decades, the world has seen a really startling increase in the number of children and adults with peanut and nut allergies. What is going on here? How can it be possible that a common ingredient and a good source of nutrition can make so many people very seriously ill? There are more than 3 million Americans living with a peanut allergy, a colossal number. In Britain, it is estimated that one in fifty children now has an allergy to nuts, a rate which has doubled in a decade and which means there are now a quarter of a million young sufferers.

Peanuts are among the most common allergy-causing foods, and they often find their way into things you wouldn't imagine had any trace of them. Food is cooked in peanut oil; stews are sometimes thickened with it. In fact, peanuts aren't a true nut at all but are actually classified as a legume (in the same family as pulses such as peas and lentils). People can also be allergic to tree nuts, such as almonds, walnuts, pecans, cashews – and even sunflower and sesame seeds.

What is happening in the body?

When a person with a nut or peanut allergy eats the substance, even a miniscule amount of it, the immune system reacts very badly. No one is sure why nuts should trigger this particular reaction, but as explained in Chapter 1 (see page 18), the allergic response means that the antibody IgE is produced and triggers the release of a host of other chemicals. These go into overdrive to protect the body, but actually inflame other organs.

The production of these chemicals can affect the respiratory system, gastrointestinal tract, the skin and the cardiovascular system – causing symptoms such as wheezing, nausea, headache, stomach-ache and itchy rashes. The symptoms, which may occur immediately or take place a few hours later, affect:

- The skin – in the form of red, bumpy rashes (hives), eczema, or redness and widespread swelling under the skin and around the mouth caused by fluid escaping from the blood vessels into the tissues.

- The gastrointestinal tract – in the form of belly cramps, diarrhoea, nausea or vomiting.

- The respiratory tract – symptoms can range from a runny nose, itchy, watery eyes and sneezing to difficulty in breathing, swallowing or speaking and the triggering of asthma with coughing and wheezing.

- The heart – rapid pulse, palpitations.

While some people may just have a mild reaction, such as itchy skin, for others it is much more serious and it can cause a reaction known as anaphylactic shock. Anaphylaxis is a sudden, potentially fatal allergic reaction which can cause blood pressure to drop suddenly, the airways to narrow and the tongue to swell, resulting in serious breathing difficulty, loss of consciousness, and, in some cases, even death. It usually occurs minutes after exposure to a triggering substance, such as a peanut, but some reactions may be delayed by as long as four hours.

A few, very unfortunate sufferers are so acutely sensitive that just by being in the same room as nuts and breathing in small particles, they can suffer a reaction. This has prompted many restaurants and some airlines to stop serving peanuts altogether.

For reasons that are not fully understood, a nut allergy doesn't seem to work in the same way as a dairy allergy, which you can grow out of over time. With nuts and peanuts, it tends to be for life. Over time, sufferers and their families learn how to avoid what is making them so ill and food manufacturers are getting more responsible about not including nuts in their products – or at least labelling them if they are included.

Identifying a nut allergy

If you suspect that you or your child have a nut allergy, it is important to see a specialist for testing. You will be asked questions about why you suspect it and what the reactions have been and whether there is a history of allergies in the family. You are likely to be given a skin-prick test, which will involve placing a liquid extract of nut or peanut onto the skin, pricking it and seeing if there is a reaction.

Some doctors may also take a blood sample and send it to a lab where it will be mixed with some of the suspected allergen and checked for IgE antibodies. If the results of these tests are still unclear, a food challenge may be needed for final diagnosis (this test is done only in certain cases). During this test, a person might be given gradually increasing amounts of nuts or peanuts to eat while being watched for symptoms by the doctor. This test should only be performed in a doctor's surgery or hospital that has access to full medical care. Allergy specialists usually avoid giving this test to people who have experienced a severe reaction to nuts or peanuts in the past.

Treatment

The only really successful way to treat a nut or peanut allergy is through complete avoidance. However, this means a lot more than just simply not eating nuts. It involves the person not even touching them or being around people who are eating them. It also involves not eating any food where there is the slightest suspicion that it may contain nuts in the ingredients. In some cases, miniscule amounts of nuts and peanuts can find their way into foods that shouldn't contain them. This may be the case if a food product is made in a place that manufactures other products which do contain nuts.

It is essential to avoid any foods you're not sure about, such as baked goods, desserts, or other products that you haven't prepared yourself, or for which you don't know the ingredients. It's also possible that a food that doesn't contain nut ingredients may have come into contact with nuts or peanuts if it's produced in a factory that also processes these ingredients (this is called cross-contamination). Some factories may use the same equipment for nuts or peanuts as they do for products that don't contain them, so tiny amounts of the allergen could be transferred to other foods.

Always read the label

The best way to be sure a food is nut free is to read the label. As of January 2006, manufacturers of foods sold in the United States have to list on their labels whether a food contains – or may contain – any of the most common allergens. The same is true for the UK and across the EU. But there are all kinds of flaws in the labelling system. Using the catch-all phrase 'may contain' allows manufacturers to cover themselves in case an ingredient, such as a nut, has slipped through the production process. The danger is that some consumers may start to ignore this very general warning when there is actually a real risk of contamination. Also, companies do not have to mention any ingredients that are used at the first stage of the manufacturing process, before the food reaches them, such as wheat flour added to spices.

In an emergency

For anyone who has had a serious reaction to a nut or peanut, it is essential to carry with you at all times emergency medication, which comes in the form of a syringe known as an EpiPen or Anapen. When you become ill, this device can deliver into your body a shot of adrenaline (also known as epinephrine). It can also be taken in the form of an inhaler, but this is not a substitute for the syringe. The adrenaline stops the airways narrowing further, prevents the fall in blood pressure and starts to stop some of the allergic response.

To apply the medication, the syringe needs to be jabbed firmly into the muscle of the thigh. It is easy to use but important that patients are shown how and when to use it by medical staff, who can also get you to practise using a dummy injector. Anyone with a heart condition should talk to their doctor about suitability as adrenaline can affect the heart.

If it is a child who has the allergy, it is imperative that adrenaline is kept at the school and even at the houses of their close circle of friends.

In the event of an emergency where you have to use the medication, you should always go straight to a hospital or doctor so that they can give you additional treatment if necessary. Some specialists like to observe patients for up to eight hours afterwards because there can be further symptoms after the initial attack.

Living with the allergy

- Avoid eating at self-service counters or buffets where people may put spoons in and out of different bowls, risking cross-contamination.

- If you ask a waiter or cook if the food is prepared without using nuts or nut oil, and they don't seem sure, don't eat it.

- Make your own snacks and lunches to take to other people's houses, parties, school, and on field trips so you always have 'safe' food.

- In the case of a child, be sure everyone at school – from the head teacher and staff to friends and classmates – knows about the food allergy. The school should make every attempt to ensure that the lunch room is a nut-free area. If they don't, you'll have to ask for a separate room.

- Encourage friends and family to wash their hands with soap after meals. Just rinsing hands with water alone or using an alcohol-based hand sanitiser will not remove all nut or peanut residues.

- Avoid fried foods (especially in restaurants and fast-food places) that may be made with peanut oil or may contain hidden peanuts or nuts.

- Teach close friends to recognise the signs of anaphylaxis and show them how to help you.

- If going on holiday, get a written statement to explain your condition in the correct language to staff in the hotel or restaurant.

• Fish allergy

Fish allergy can often cause severe reactions, including anaphylactic shock. Adults are more likely to be allergic to fish and shellfish than children, probably because adults will have eaten these foods more often.

People who are allergic to one type of fish, such as cod, often react to other types of fish such as hake, haddock, mackerel and whiting as well. This is because the allergens in these fish are quite similar. Avoidance is the only real solution and, again, sufferers should read the labels very carefully and ask the right questions in restaurants.

Someone with a fish allergy could also have an allergic reaction to fish-oil supplements. It is the protein in the food that triggers a reaction and some of that protein could be present in the oil. The reaction will depend on the person's sensitivity to the protein and also the amount of it in the supplement itself. When in doubt, it is best to avoid taking such supplements altogether.

122

Food intolerance

There is growing evidence to suggest that quite a lot of people have an intolerance to one or more groups of food. The Digestive Disorders Foundation in the UK, a reputable patient organisation, puts the number who may suffer an intolerance at around 3 per cent but the reality is that no one can accurately state the true prevalence (rate within a population) because it is so difficult to diagnose.

Allergy specialists and others can point to a number of studies which suggest that it is very real indeed, for example, studies looking at migraine patients have linked the condition back to food. The controversy surrounding the subject of food intolerance should have prompted more in-depth clinical trials but, so far, it has not. However, the current state of the scientific investigation into the problem is well laid out in the book *Food Allergy and Intolerance* by Professor Jonathan Brostoff and Linda Gamlin.

The good news is that there are definite signs that things are changing. Family doctors are becoming more aware of the nature of food intolerance and are able to offer sound advice. In Britain, with its deplorable lack of allergy specialists, it is hard to get proper specialist help through the National Health Service so many patients are forced to go private but, actually, it is possible to help yourself. The first stage is to go on an elimination diet, which should not be done without prior discussion with your doctor. This involves cutting out food groups that could possibly cause a reaction and seeing if this produces a symptom-free state. If it does, then the different food groups are then individually reintroduced, each in their pure form, to pinpoint exactly which ones are causing the symptoms. If problem foods are identified, they should then be cut out completely. For a more detailed explanation on how to follow an elimination diet, see pages 131–134.

• The symptoms

How do you know if you have a food intolerance? One of the great problems with this condition – and one of the reasons why it is often derided by doctors – is that no two people will have the same symptoms and, also they may change over time. Very often, these symptoms can be caused by other illnesses, so it is very important that you have them checked out by your GP.

Below are the symptoms which are commonly associated with food intolerance:

*   Migraines, or severe headaches

*   Bouts of diarrhoea, sometimes with wind

*   Constipation

*   Nausea, indigestion

*   Joint pain

*   A runny nose

*   Feeling constantly tired and run-down

*   In children, problems such as persistent stomach-ache or glue ear

*   In babies, some doctors think that colic can be a reaction to food, even including the tiny amount of cow's milk that the mother is eating, and may be coming through the breast milk

Many patients opt for self-diagnosis and cut out a particular substance, such as wheat, from their diet in the belief that it will help them. There is nothing harmful about this as long as you still maintain a fully balanced diet. But before you rush into diagnosing yourself with a particular intolerance, it is extremely important that you talk to your doctor about the symptoms you've been experiencing. Receiving professional help in this area is very important and you may well not get to the root of the problem without it.

• Why the reaction?

Several factors may cause a person to have an adverse reaction to a particular food. Sometimes the body is reacting to chemicals that are found naturally in foods such as cheese or eggs. But in some cases, it is the additives in the foods that are causing the problems.

Many patients can trace back the beginning of their problems to a particular spell of illness and a number of specialists have linked food intolerances to the use of antibiotics, which can upset the natural balance of gut flora, the collection of good bacteria and yeasts which live in our intestines.

An antibiotic kills bacteria when you have an infection, but they are not very discriminating – they tend to wipe out the good as well as the bad bugs. So it is very common after taking a course of antibiotics to suffer from a spell of diarrhoea as the gut struggles to right itself. It is known, for example, that following a hysterectomy, many women suffer from these disturbances that can be painful and distressing.

Doctors who deal a lot with food intolerance cases say that many patients will trace the beginnings of their problems back to a spell of bad diarrhoea, and that their health has never seemed the same afterwards. One possibility is that the illness has made the gut leaky, so that tiny fragments of proteins escape the normal digestion process and end up in the bloodstream, where they set up a reaction. One of the strangest things about these intolerances is that patients often crave the very food that makes them ill.

• Carbohydrate intolerance

Some people cannot digest certain carbohydrates, compounds that provide us with most of the energy required for a healthy diet. Carbohydrates exist as simple sugars (sucrose, glucose, fructose and lactose) or as glucose polymers (complex carbohydrates), such as glycogen and cellulose. In many intolerance cases, individuals have problems digesting a simple sugar carbohydrate called lactose (milk sugar). In other cases, the problem involves the digestion of sugars often found in fruit juices.

Lactose intolerance occurs when an individual is deficient in lactase, an intestinal enzyme which the body needs to digest the lactose in milk and other dairy products. As a result, the undigested lactose remains in the intestines, causing abdominal cramps, bloating and diarrhoea.

Babies are usually born with higher levels of lactase, so lactose intolerance usually only begins after the age of about two, as the body begins to produce less of the enzyme. However, many people don't experience symptoms until they're much older. A temporary lactase deficiency may follow gastroenteritis, especially in children.

The condition is far more common in certain countries and ethnic groups than in others. In areas where milk is not usually part of the diet, a much greater number of people are affected. That is why in South America, Africa and Asia, more than 50 per cent of the population are intolerant to lactose, rising to nearly 100 per cent in some parts of Asia. In the UK, Ireland, Northern Europe and North America, it is thought that about 5 per cent of the adult population have this condition.

125

Digestive diseases or injuries to the small intestine can sometimes cause lactose intolerance, because damage to the lining of the small intestine may reduce the amount of lactase enzyme which is produced. In extremely rare cases, the condition can be inherited.

The bad news is that milk from all animals, including cows, goats, sheep and humans, contains lactose. There is no medical treatment for lactose intolerance, but symptoms can be avoided by controlling the amount in the diet. Some adults can tolerate just a small amount without reacting and many people switch to soya milk, although some are allergic to this too.

case study ───────────────────────────────────

Julia Reid couldn't understand why it was becoming so hard to breastfeed her baby, Calum. After every feed, he would start to vomit a good deal more than seemed natural. She began to worry that he wasn't going to put on weight, and that he seemed to be in pain after a feed.

Her GP initially told her that it was probably colic, and she tried to give him some stomach-soothing medication. 'It didn't really help, and then I began to wonder what was wrong.' But then she suspected it might be a form of milk allergy and the GP agreed that this was a possibility.

The vomiting after food, known as reflux, was a sign that the stomach couldn't tolerate the lactose in the milk. Julia was lucky enough to be sent to a specialist paediatrician in Liverpool, who carried out allergy tests on Calum, then just six months old.

The test results came back as not having a milk allergy, but the doctors told her that the tests were not always accurate and that the details Julia gave them pointed to some form of allergy or intolerance. Julia carried on breastfeeding because it was important that he still received the nutrients, but then started to wean him at five months, keeping him off dairy products. The vomiting stopped, and it seemed the introduction of solids helped him keep the food down.

'A year later, I tried him on a dairy product and he was absolutely fine, so I suppose it was something which he grew out of,' said Julia, a university lecturer from Leeds. She has since discovered that reflux is very common, and often put down to colic when it may be something more. Meanwhile, her son seems to be allergic to eggs and nuts, so she has to be careful to ensure that he doesn't take in these foods by accident.

case study 💬

• Soya intolerance

Although soya intolerance may not be as common as an intolerance to dairy products, it does appear to be on the increase. This is probably due to the fact that soya is now being added to so many foods, so young babies are exposed to it at a much earlier age than would otherwise be the case.

Many doctors define it as an allergy rather than an intolerance because it can cause serious symptoms including rashes, diarrhoea, vomiting, stomach cramps and breathing difficulties. In rare cases, it can even lead to anaphylactic shock. It is a common childhood allergy and most children grow out of it by the age of two, but occasionally adults are allergic to soya.

Some people with soya allergy might also react to milk.

According to the UK's food regulator, the Food Standards Agency, soya is used as an ingredient in lots of food products, including some bakery goods, sweets, drinks, breakfast cereals, ice cream, margarine, pasta and processed meats. Soya flour is used to increase the shelf life of many products and to improve the colour of pastry crusts. Textured soya protein is used as a meat substitute and to improve the consistency of meat products.

Since November 2005, food labelling rules require pre-packed food sold in the UK, or the rest of the European Union (EU), to show clearly on the label if it contains soya (or if one of its ingredients contains it). But you have to remember that there could still be foods on the shelves that were produced before this date.

• Alcohol intolerance

An alcohol intolerance also involves a deficiency of an enzyme, this case aldehyde dehydrogenase, which is needed to break down alcohol. Drinking even small amounts can make affected people feel unwell.

• Additives

Some people have adverse reactions to chemical preservatives and additives contained in many foods. Particular culprits include sulphites, benzoates, salicylates, monosodium glutamate, caffeine, aspartame and tartrazine. Sulphites, in particular, which are sulphur-based and have been used since ancient times to preserve food, are now increasingly implicated in food intolerances. Sulphites are found in:

*   Dried fruit

*   Jam

*   Shellfish

*   Delicatessen meat

*   White wine

*   Frozen potatoes and chips

How one woman changed a supermarket

Patricia Wheway sometimes felt like tearing her hair out. She had given up a senior management job with a British company in order to become a full-time mother but looking after her five year old, George, was not easy. He had epilepsy, learning difficulties and bowel problems and Patricia realised he was also reacting badly to cow's milk, gluten and artificial additives.

Hours of her day would go into preparing food that he could eat without becoming ill. In her frustration, she wrote to the chief executive of one of the major UK supermarkets, Tesco. She sent Sir Terry Leahy a business plan for the kinds of allergy food that any proper supermarket should have on its shelves. She was amazed when he wrote back, asking to meet her and then gave her a job of making it happen.

In 2002, Tesco launched its *Free From* range which prompted most of the other major supermarkets to follow suit. Now Patricia works as the company's brand manager and has also developed an additive-free *Tesco Kids* range. She is so glad she took that initial step.

'When I was at home, desperately researching how to get the right foods for George, I remember thinking, "Is this my life? Is this all there is?" But if something bad or dramatic happens to you, you can either become a victim and say, "Why me?" or you can say, "What can I do to beat it?" All I know is that for me, personally, I knew I had to do something to get myself out of this situation. I had ideas about what supermarkets should be doing for children like George. I told some friends and they suggested I contact Tesco since they were so big on being customer-orientated.'

By reducing the number of artificial additives George was eating, he became less hyperactive. Once Patricia started him on a gluten-free diet, the diarrhoea stopped. He is now ten years old and is free from the problems.

All the supermarkets have had to take a crash course in how to offer products which can protect an increasing number of customers who suffer from allergies. Much of this is due to one mother refusing to accept the status quo and persuading people that things had to change.

• Coeliac disease

For patients with this condition, simply eating a piece of toast can be profoundly painful. This lifelong disorder is caused by an intolerance to gluten, the protein found in wheat and a few other grains. What happens is that the proteins in the gluten actually damage the tiny finger-like projections, known as villi, that line the small intestine. When the villi are damaged, it prevents the normal absorption of food constituents, particularly fats, and this leads to both diarrhoea and serious weight loss due to malnutrition.

Coeliac disease, which occurs in around one in every hundred people in Britain, involves an immune response. Sufferers develop antibodies against one of their own proteins, an enzyme called tissue-transglutaminase. The job of this enzyme, found in the intestine, is to assist with the breakdown of gluten.

Needless to say, it is extremely important to get this condition diagnosed as soon as possible because of the risk of malnutrition and the serious effects it can have. A specialised blood test can tell doctors whether the patient is likely to have Coeliac disease and they may also need to go to hospital for an intestinal biopsy, to have it confirmed by a specialist. There is no cure for the condition – but it can be controlled by following a gluten-free diet and, thankfully, there are now quite a few companies which offer a range of such foods.

129

• Irritable bowel syndrome

The word 'syndrome' is used by doctors to describe a condition that has a whole collection of symptoms, which is very much the case with irritable bowel syndrome (IBS), the two most common being cramping pains in the abdomen and irregular bowel habits. Sometimes sufferers find they have to get to the toilet fast, but often they also experience bouts of constipation. Life, in short, becomes painful and difficult as the bowel begins to dictate so much of your life – not just your toilet habits, but your moods, your sleeping patterns and your energy levels.

Doctors believe that IBS is probably the most common disorder of the digestive system. Around one-third of the population experience symptoms from time to time and women are slightly more affected than men. The usual age of onset is between twenty and forty and, once diagnosed, it is usual to be referred to a specialist.

We still don't know much about the causes of the condition, but it is clear that it is not an allergy to food. There is some evidence that it starts after a period when patients have been eating very irregularly or when they have had a bad dose of food poisoning or gastroenteritis. Stress seems to make the symptoms worse but it does with many illnesses, so that is hardly surprising.

Treatment for IBS

Doctors may need to give you a blood test to rule out anaemia, or lack of iron, to make sure that your other organs are working properly and also to rule out any inflammation of the bowel.

If it is thought that your symptoms are being caused by something you are eating, the doctor may recommend an exclusion or elimination diet (see opposite). If the symptoms subsequently improve, then you can add specific foods back into the diet until the one that is causing you problems is identified. If constipation is a particular problem, it may mean gradually increasing your fibre intake, or alternatively reducing it if you suffer from frequent bouts of diarrhoea or bloating.

130

There are now drug therapies available to help to reduce the painful bowel spasms associated with IBS, however they don't necessarily benefit everyone. Exercise can help reduce attacks as it helps tone up the stomach muscles and prevents the intestine from swelling up so much. Regular exercise will also help to alleviate any stress.

• Finding solutions to food intolerance

Angela from Milwaukee, USA, has suffered from stomach cramps since she was a child. But now, at the age of 27, she feels for the first time that she has some control over her life. However, it has been a long, slow process.

'I suppose that since I was a child, I've had at least one painful attack a week,' she explains. 'It all began to improve in 2001, when I decided to stop eating wheat. It was really hard, as I loved pasta and pizza, but it helped so much.

'However, I was still getting cramps, although much less regularly over the following year, so I decided to cut out dairy too. This was really difficult too but I ate much more fruit and vegetables and switched to soya, which I could tolerate. It just meant I had to spend a lot more time planning my meals.

'One thing that has really gone is the craving for pizza – it was terrible at first but now I don't miss it at all. I still get the odd cramps and bouts of diarrhoea but it really doesn't hurt in the way it did.

'A lot of people feel too embarrassed to talk about their problems but it's amazing how interested people are – and they'll often end up telling you about their own experiences. I do miss being able to eat out but you get used to it – instead I go to the cinema a lot more now.'

Angela found her own solutions to her problems by simply cutting out certain food groups – and watching to see if it made a difference to her symptoms.

This kind of elimination diet is a very common way of trying to find a solution to the pain and discomfort, but it doesn't work for everyone and can be a very long and frustrating process. You can end up cutting out foodstuffs and still be left with symptoms that may be caused by another aspect of your diet.

The elimination diet

This type of eating plan involves removing specific foods or ingredients from your diet that you and your doctor suspect may be causing symptoms. It is always important to talk to your doctor before embarking on any such plan. It's not a quick fix and you need to prepare for this in several ways.

131

- Talk to your friends or family about what you are doing so that they aren't surprised when you turn down going out for a meal or having a drink in the evening.

- Start to read food labels carefully and work out what you can and can't eat.

- Keep a symptoms diary before you begin the diet, to chronicle what you are experiencing. This will produce a useful guide to compare with the symptoms you have once you are on the diet.

- A food diary is also necessary, in which you record each day the foods you are eating. This is important, because you need to be disciplined and this will produce an accurate record which will be useful later on.

- At the beginning of this diet, you are going to feel tired and lacking in energy. Make sure you don't have any big work commitments that might be compromised by being on the diet.

- While following this diet, make sure you are eating other foods that provide the same nutrients as those you've eliminated (for example, try tofu-based foods instead of dairy products). Talk this through with your doctor. If you have the help of a dietitian, they can advise you on how to plan meals that are healthy and nutritious without including the potentially allergenic foods.

It is important to remember that this kind of regime is not suitable for anyone with a true allergy, such as an allergy to nuts. It can provoke a strong and dangerous reaction. Doctors advise that if you have ever had a very bad reaction to a food, such as violent sickness, you should steer clear of this course of action. Nor is this diet suitable for people with particular conditions, such as Crohn's disease or atopic eczema.

Some experts believe that before beginning an elimination diet, it's a good idea to start with a healthy eating regime, in which you exclude the drinks and foods that are full of additives and stimulants that can commonly cause problems. This doesn't mean cutting out wheat and eggs, for example, but items such as coffee, alcohol and very sugary foods. Some people like to begin on this basis, spending a month really cutting down on the 'bad' unhealthy foods to find out whether this actually lessens their symptoms. Starting off in this way can also make it easier to adjust to the changes before going onto the full-blown elimination diet.

How to begin

Once you embark on this diet, you have to exclude all the foods that you would normally eat regularly, such as cheese, bread, butter or oranges. Make a list of what you eat in the average week and then work out a list of foods that you don't often touch.

If, for example, you normally eat a lot of cabbage, you have to exclude foods that are closely related, such as broccoli or Brussels sprouts. With oranges, you might exclude lemon and grapefruit as they are also citrus fruits.

It's not easy to 'outlaw' all your favourite foods, but you should be able to find at least ten other foods that you think you will be able to eat over a period of at least seven to ten days. They should include the following:

Fruits and vegetables These should not be the ones you eat regularly. Look at mangoes, pears, nectarines, leeks, parsnips and pumpkin.

Starch As you are excluding bread and wheat, this becomes harder, but you need to include some starch. Think of yams and the more unusual products such as sago, millet or buckwheat, which can be delicious.

Meat Go for meats you don't normally try such as venison or pheasant. Unfortunately for vegetarians, both soya and quorn must be avoided but put nuts on the list as a source of protein. Try to vary the varieties you eat to avoid consuming the ones that are normally part of your diet.

What you cannot include in your diet:

- Herbs, spices and flavourings, including salt

- Coffee, tea, alcohol and all soft drinks

- Sugar – and all things containing sugar

- No tinned or packaged food – buy it raw and prepare it yourself

- All the foods you would normally eat, especially anything containing wheat and dairy

133

The first week

Going on this diet is not easy, but you have to see it as a means to an end – the understanding of what it is that makes you ill. During the first seven days, you will feel tired and lethargic as your body reacts to the big change in your eating habits. You may find the symptoms actually worsen over this period. Many people suffer headaches or a migraine, so be prepared for this first week to be hard. Try not to rely on any one food every single day and vary what you eat as much as possible. After day six or seven, you should start to feel slightly better. Remember to keep a full diary of both your symptoms and your diet so that you can compare the changes later.

If you do not experience any change in your symptoms after a week to ten days, food is probably not causing your problems and, therefore, you should not go onto the next stage. Again, make sure you talk fully to your doctor about this.

Reintroducing foods

By now, you should have become used to keeping a full diary each day about your eating patterns and your symptoms. This becomes crucial in the next phase, which is about reintroducing different food groups back into the diet. You should allow about two months for this stage and it has to be done methodically, or it won't work.

For the first two weeks, start to eat the foods which you enjoy but are not the mainstay of your normal diet. This is likely to be fruit and vegetables. It can also include certain meats such as chicken.

Test one new food each day, and make sure you don't over-eat. Record any reaction to the food which might not happen immediately, but some hours afterwards. One of the difficulties is that you may suffer a bowel problem, such as diarrhoea, up to forty-eight hours later and so you need to keep an accurate record. If this happens, and you are unsure which food caused it, you should drop all the foods that you suspect, and reintroduce them later for a three-day period. In this situation, you eat some of that food daily for three days and if you have no reaction to it, you know it is not the cause of the problems.

Wheat and milk products should be left until the end. Reintroduce these slowly, when you've built up your diet into a more normal pattern, and then eat the wheat-based products over three days to see if there is a reaction. Doctors suggest that you shouldn't start with bread, because it contains yeast – which can cause an intolerance – and instead look at reintroducing a cereal.

The final stage

It is possible that food intolerances are caused by the common additives found in food. Towards the end of the eight-week period, it is sensible to introduce packaged foods to see if these are causing a reaction. Just make sure that they contain the ingredients that you have already found safe, rather than reintroducing a new food as well as the additives.

The diet shouldn't go on for more than eight weeks. If you still haven't had symptoms back, you can go onto three-day testing, where you eat some of the foods each day for three days. But if you reintroduce all the foods and there are no symptoms, you need to talk to your doctor or a dietitian about what to do next.

What next?

For anyone who has successfully identified the food group that is making them ill, the usual habit is to cut it out completely. The strange aspect of food intolerances is that you can grow out of them. Possibly, within a year, you may find yourself able to eat something safely again, but even if this is the case it is still a good idea to limit amounts and not to over-indulge.

• Food intolerances and children

There are a growing number of parents who believe their children may have a food intolerance, but finding out what it is – or if it even exists – is no easy matter. Children can develop stomach-aches for a host of reasons, including depression or hyperactivity, and it is dangerous to cut out major food groups while maintaining a balanced diet.

If you do believe your child has developed a food intolerance, it is good to talk to your doctor about it first, in case he or she thinks that some tests may be needed. In some, rare cases children are born with metabolic abnormalities which means they become ill if they eat certain types of food. These youngsters are missing some of the enzymes needed to process food, possibly due to genetic flaws. One of the most common is primary lactase deficiency, a lifelong condition developed as a baby which means that the child cannot properly absorb the sugar coming from the milk.

Some hospitals may conduct a 'food challenge' test if they need to determine that a food allergy exists or to confirm a suspected food allergy. A sample of the suspected offending food is given to the person unknowingly. The suspected offending food may be mixed with another food or may be disguised as an ingredient in another food. These food preparation techniques are used to prevent undue influence on the outcome of the test (if the person recognises the food by sight or taste). Another method is to have the person take a capsule containing the allergen.

This test is given under strict supervision because of the dangers of reaction – and this would never be attempted on anyone with a history of severe reactions. After eating the food or taking the capsule, the person is monitored to see if a reaction occurs.

PART THREE
MANAGING ALLERGIES

CHAPTER TEN
DIAGNOSIS

Identifying your allergy

Once you think you have developed an allergy, it is important to go and see your doctor, who will hopefully be sympathetic and want to get to the bottom of whatever is causing you or your child to feel ill. However, for many people, simply getting a proper diagnosis is not always easy.

Identifying an allergy is not like identifying cancer or heart disease. There is no one test or scan that can be performed to give patients a definitive answer. This is why it is crucially important that anyone who thinks they may have an allergy knows all about the different tests available. To a certain extent, you have to become an expert in the field even before you know whether you've got a particular sensitivity to a chemical or a food or not.

Karen Jones (not her real name) spent nearly a year trying to find out what was causing a range of problems for her ten-year-old daughter, Sarah.

 case study ————————————————————

My husband and I began to feel that something wasn't right with Sarah. She seemed extremely lethargic, more than a ten year old should be and she had a constant runny nose. Sometimes she would wake up in the morning and her eyes would be really puffy.

'We thought at first it was hayfever, so we dosed her up with an over-the-counter medication and told her school about it, but the syrup didn't work. A friend of ours then recommended that we saw a private kinesiologist (who uses a diagnostic technique that works on the principle that each muscle in the body is related to an internal organ). It cost us a lot but we felt we had no choice. This man did some tests and told us that she was allergic to wheat and citrus fruit. So we radically changed her diet but Sarah still had this constant cold and actually seemed to get more run down, not less.

'In the end, my mum suggested that we see the GP and try to get her referred to a specialist. The GP was great and was able to perform a skin-prick test which showed that Sarah had an allergy to cat dander – so all the time it was our pet that was causing her problems. I felt very bad that we hadn't thought about this sooner and I wish I had gone to see the doctor earlier but, somehow, I thought it was my job to sort it out.

'We re-homed our cat and put Sarah back on to a normal diet and her problems cleared up quickly. I notice that she still does start to go puffy around the eyes if she goes to a friend's house who has a cat, so I now ask the parents in advance to keep the animals out of the room and we try to have her friends over to our house instead. The solution turned out to be fairly simple once we got to the right person.'

case study

The first port of call for anyone who suspects they may have an allergy should be their family doctor. Don't be lured by the many internet sites offering quick diagnoses – go for the more reliable route. Your doctor should take a clinical history from you, asking about your symptoms, details of when they occur and any other relevant information such as whether anyone else in the family has an allergy.

In the UK, there is a huge lack of specialist allergy services, to the point where it is really a national scandal. Despite the fact that one in three people in the UK may suffer from an allergy during their lifetime, there are only three paediatric allergy specialists for the whole country and only ninety allergy clinics altogether. This is because the NHS has failed to invest in these services and instead leaves it to individuals like Karen Jones to muddle through. If you do need to see a specialist, you are likely to be put on a waiting list that could mean it is several months before you see someone.

But don't be put off by the shortage of specialist care. It is still possible for you to have the tests you or your child needs if you are persistent enough. And if you are offered the chance to go on the waiting list, take it. It is always better to see a specialist if you can, because they are the people who really have an in-depth knowledge of your condition. For details of allergy specialists, see Useful Websites, pages 188–189).

The different means of diagnosis   141

• Skin-prick test

This test is most commonly performed on the forearm, although the back is also sometimes used. The arm is first cleaned with an alcohol wipe, then a drop of commercially-produced allergen extract is placed onto the marked area of skin. Using a sterile lancet (needle), a tiny prick through the drop is made. This doesn't hurt, but allows a small amount of the allergen to enter the skin. If you have a reaction, a small lump like a mosquito bite will appear at the site of testing within fifteen to twenty minutes. This is known as a weal and will fade within a few hours. But the larger the weal, the more serious your allergy.

There are a whole range of allergens that can be tested in this way. For patients who suspect they have hayfever or asthma, testing usually includes allergens such as house-dust mite, cat and dog dander, spores from mould, and particular grasses, weeds and tree pollens. Testing can also be used to confirm suspected food allergy and stinging insect venom allergy.

A variation on this is the scratch test, where instead of the skin being pricked with a lancet, a scratch is made and the allergen-containing liquid poured over it. However, some doctors feel that this method is slightly less reliable.

Skin-prick testing doesn't work for all allergens. It is not an accurate way of diagnosing reactions to aspirin or food additives. Nor is it 100 per cent reliable and, occasionally, it can produce false results. It should, however, be performed on all patients suspected of suffering from severe episodic or persistent asthma, as well as in those with suspected hayfever, or suspected allergic reactions to stinging venomous insects or particular foods.

There are no age limitations for skin testing, although the very young and the elderly may have diminished reactions and those less than two years old are only occasionally sensitised to inhaled allergens anyway. It is also not advisable for pregnant women because if they suffer a severe allergic reaction as a result of the test, they could experience womb contractions.

• Blood test

This test will measure the amount of immunoglobulin E antibodies (IgE) in the blood (the antibody responsible for the allergic reaction, see page 18). A sample of blood is taken and sent to a specialist laboratory for what is known as the RAST (Radio-allergosorbent Test) or CAP-RAST test. For example, if you have a suspected allergy to house-dust mite, the level of house-dust mite IgE will be raised. The result is then graded 0 to 6, depending on the level of that particular IgE in the blood. Over 400 different allergens can be tested for in this way.

This type of testing is particularly useful in certain cases, such as severe eczema all over the body, where an allergy skin test cannot be done. For diagnosis of milk, egg, wheat, peanut or fish allergy, the CAP-RAST test may also be more useful than skin tests.

However, there can be a danger of false positives, particularly for food allergies, where a patient tests positive for an allergen they are not allergic to. Patients with eczema have very high levels of IgE and if they are being tested for a food allergy, a false positive result can occur. This is because there is so much IgE present in the blood sample that it shows up as a positive result for foods that the person is not allergic to. There is also the danger that foods with similar protein structures may cross-react, resulting in false positive results.

• Patch test

This test is used to diagnose delayed allergic reactions such as contact dermatitis, which affects the skin (see Chapter Eight, Contact Dermatitis). It should be done on a skin site where the dermatitis is not apparent and can be very useful for people who are suffering from unexplained rashes or blisters. The test involves placing the various known allergens, which are mixed with a non-allergic material, directly onto the skin. They are then held in place with special adhesive tape and are left for forty-eight hours. The skin is then examined by a doctor, who will see if there has been any kind of response to the allergen. This is a good way of determining whether you might have an allergy to rubber, nickel, lanolin, various dyes, cosmetics, preservatives and medication.

The dermatologist will suggest which allergens you should be tested for, partly based on the information you have supplied about the substances you commonly come into contact with. One such patch test is known as the European Standard Battery, which consists of the commonest allergens that cause 85 per cent of all allergic skin reactions. The resulting allergic response is then given a score, which can range from being 'doubtful', where there is only a very mild redness, to 'positive' where the skin has become intensely red and swollen, with blisters appearing.

• Challenge test

This test is performed in hospital and involves medical staff introducing the suspected allergen directly into the nose, mouth, lung or eye to see if they can provoke, and measure, an allergic reaction. It is the most accurate way to test for food allergies, but it is not simple or fast.

To start with, the patient is often given a 'dummy' substance which is hidden in another food or spray and is completely harmless. This is so that doctors can see whether or not the patient is truly reacting to the allergen because, for some patients, simply thinking about the allergen can provoke a reaction.

For a suspected food allergy, staff may use the Double Blind Placebo Controlled Food Challenge (DBPCFC) test. The offending food is concealed in a capsule or broth and, under careful supervision, is given to the patient to see if they react to it. This must only be done in a specialist allergy clinic which has full resuscitation equipment available because of the risks of a patient going into anaphylactic shock (see page 178).

Sometimes shorter 'open challenges' are performed where the patient is aware of what they are eating. This is a test where the patient is asked to eat a suspect food that is not disguised in any way, so they know exactly what they are eating. This can be used where patients have shown no signs of reaction in a previous test, and the doctor then asks the patient to eat a standard portion of the suspected food to double check there is no allergy. The open challenge is also used to test a food that produced a positive RAST or skin-prick test result, but which through the patient's history has never been thought to cause a problem.

Open challenges do carry the potential risk of causing an allergic reaction and should only be performed with proper medical supervision.

When it comes to a food intolerance, the only really reliable way of achieving a conclusive result is to go on an elimination diet, (see pages 131–134). However, this takes a lot of time and effort, which is why many people have sought out other methods. Unfortunately, many of the alternative methods don't work. A brief outline of some of those available follows, but it is important to talk to your doctor before using any of them.

Alternative testing

There is now an enormous market in alternative testing for allergies simply because patients are so desperate to find a diagnosis. However, some practitioners perform tests that have not been shown to have an acceptable degree of diagnostic reliability. According to the British Society for Allergy and Clinical Immunology (the association representing mainstream NHS specialists who promote allergy clinics and better treatment for patients), they shouldn't be relied on for allergy diagnostic purposes because they are of an inferior nature.

Dr Adrian Morris, a GP in the UK with over fourteen years of allergy experience, who runs a clinic in Surrey, points out: 'These unvalidated tests are promoted by complementary and alternative medicine (CAM) practitioners. Superficially, many of these tests sound plausible, but are based on unproven theories and explained with simplistic physiology. Most of these tests diagnose non-existent illnesses, are a waste of money and divert attention from actual allergies thus delaying conventional treatment that offers genuine allergy relief.' If you want to understand more about these claims and why they remain unvalidated, go to Dr Morris' website (www.allergy-clinic.co.uk) and read the papers for yourself.

• Applied kinesiology

Applied kinesiology began in 1964 and is based on the theory that signs of an organ not working properly can be detected in specific muscle weakness. This form of testing measures muscle strength in the presence of different allergens. A particular allergen is placed in the patient's mouth, or the body or in a vial in front of them, and then various muscles are tested. The patient holds out their arm and the practitioner applies a counter pressure – if the patient is unable to resist the counter pressure, the test is considered positive to that allergen. If they test 'weak', that denotes that the person has an allergy to that substance. The majority of practitioners are chiropractors, but most naturopaths, medical doctors, dentists, nutritionists and physical therapists consider this test unreliable, including the British Society for Allergy and Clinical Immunology.

These muscle-testing procedures have themselves been subjected to several well-designed controlled tests which have come to the conclusion that there is no difference in muscle response from one substance to another. The trials have demonstrated that when a placebo is given, instead of a particular allergen, the same muscle weakness is seen. Many doctors see the practice as having little substance – and the unfortunate truth is that patients end up spending a fortune on kinesiology in the hope of getting an accurate diagnosis.

• Hair analysis

Hair analysis is another questionable form of allergy testing. A strand of hair is sent away for analysis and tested for toxic levels of heavy metals such as lead, mercury and cadmium and also for mineral deficiencies, such as selenium, zinc and manganese. However, there is no reason to support the claim that high levels of these metals would have any bearing on whether or not a patient has an allergy. Numerous studies have failed to find any accuracy in hair analysis diagnosing allergies.

A variation of the hair test is called Dowsing. The dowser swings a pendulum over the hair and an allergy is diagnosed if an altered swing is noted. Again, there is little evidence to support the accuracy of this approach.

• Auriculo-cardiac reflex

Suspected allergens are placed in filter papers over the skin of the forearm. A bright light is shone through the ear lobe or back of the hand. At the same time, the pulse is taken. If the filter paper contains an allergen to which the patient is allergic, the pulse increases by twelve or more beats per minute. Again, no scientific data is available to validate this test.

• Leucocytotoxic tests

These tests, which have been around for fifty years, measure different cellular changes in the blood after the patients has been exposed to an allergen. The concept is that if the patient's white blood cells are mixed with the offending allergen, they swell. The doctor is measuring any swelling of the leukocytes and if they go beyond a certain point the patient is said to have tested positive. Studies have not been able to show that these tests are reliable markers for allergy.

• VEGA testing

146

This involves the measurement of disordered electromagnetic currents in the body to certain substances. The patient has one electrode placed over an acupuncture point and the other electrode is held while different allergens are put into a grid. A fall in the electromagnetic conductivity indicates an allergy or intolerance. According to the *British Medical Journal*, the results are very unreliable.

Britain's lamentable allergy services

Why do so many people in the UK end up going down the alternative medicine route to get their allergies diagnosed? The simple answer is because the service currently offered by the NHS is so lamentably inadequate, under-funded and under-prioritised.

There are many nurses and GPs who find themselves unable to refer patients on to specialist allergy clinics right now due to the fact that such clinics are overwhelmed by demand because there are so few of them. This pushes patients into the private sector and often into the hands of medical quacks.

In a report produced by the Royal College of Physicians in June 2003, called *Allergy: The Unmet Need*, there was a bleak warning of how poor the services were. 'There is a major shortage of allergy specialists with only six fully staffed allergy clinics in the UK that have developed, mainly around research interests. The allergy charities, along with NHS Direct, are inundated with telephone inquiries from a public desperate for help with their allergy problems. The severity of their symptoms, with attendant high morbidity [resulting in high levels of illness], has forced the public to look outside the NHS. This has led to the proliferation of dubious allergy practice in the field of complementary and alternative medicine, where unproven techniques for diagnosis and treatment are used.'

A report from the Health Select Committee of MPs made the same point a year later. The committee had recommended the development of a nationwide specialist allergy service. The government's response was that it needed more evidence before acting on the recommendations. Pamela Ewan, consultant allergist at Addenbrooke's Hospital, Cambridge, and an adviser to the Health Select Committee's inquiry into allergy, said at the time: 'A lot of allergy is multisystem, with many patients having a range of conditions, including asthma, eczema, rhinitis, and a food allergy. Full-time specialists in allergy are needed to deliver proper care to these patients, including allergy testing, appropriate treatment and anaphylaxis management, rather than their seeing different specialists, such as chest physicians, for limited elements of their care.' She called the government's request for further information a 'whitewash', and said: 'The data – including the epidemiology of allergy, the impact on patients and the health services, and evidence for the value of a specialist service – is already there.'

In 2007, the situation is no better. I asked Professor Gideon Lack at London's Guy's and St Thomas' Hospital how many paediatric (child) allergists he thought there now were in the UK. Counting on one hand, he replied: 'Three, the fourth one has just left.' Three for a country of 60 million and yet Sweden has ninety six. Guy's and St Thomas' thought they might have to advertise their allergy service when it opened up in 2006 – within months they were swamped with patients as word got round that there was some new specialist help available.

The allergy clinics run by Professor Lack and his colleagues cover not only food allergies but dermatological conditions such as eczema and chronic urticaria (itchiness), drug allergies, respiratory problems and gastroenterological problems such as reflux. Although the hospital is located in south London, it can take referrals – anywhere in the country if there is no local service available – but these have to be done via your GP.

The doctors are also hoping to hold a series of workshops for parents, working in partnership with the charity Action Against Allergy. The workshops will help parents manage their childrens' conditions both at home and when going to school. Each two-hour programme will focus on one specific condition and will give parents the chance to get answers to their questions and exchange useful ideas with others who have similar problems.

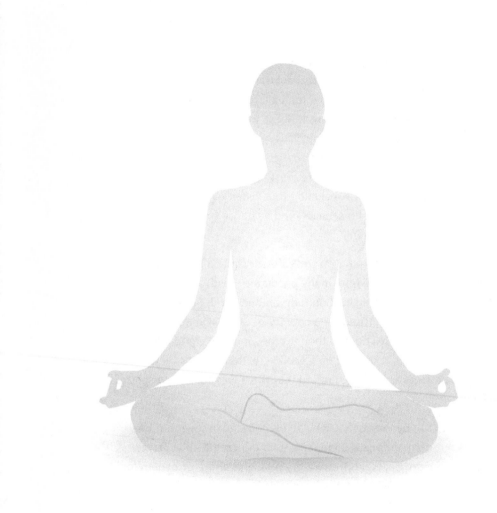

CHAPTER ELEVEN
COMPLEMENTARY THERAPIES

The use of plants for healing purposes predates human history and forms the origin of much modern medicine. Many conventional drugs originate from plant sources: a century ago, most of the few effective drugs were plant based. Examples include aspirin (from willow bark), digoxin (from foxglove), quinine (from cinchona bark), and morphine (from the opium poppy). The development of drugs from plants continues, with drug companies engaged in large scale pharmacological screening of herbs.

And now, just down the road from where I live, research is being conducted among the 1,600 species of plants native to the UK. At Kew Gardens, a famous botanical garden on the outskirts of London, its laboratory scientists are carrying out molecular tests, looking for the active compounds in different plants to see whether there is any kind of scientific basis for the claims made by herbalists about particular plants.

One of the first to show promise is figwort, a dark-leaved plant found in Northern Ireland and Norfolk, where it grows in shady woods and meadows. Nicholas Culpeper, the renowned apothecary, described it in his famous *Herbal* of 1628: 'The decoction of the herb, taken inwardly and the bruised herb applied outwardly, dissolves clotted and congealed blood within the body, comping by any wounds, bruis or fall (sic).' He added that a distilled water made from the whole plant would dry up 'hollow or corroding ulcers'.

Professor Monique Simmonds, chief plant scientist at Kew, explains how records show that, down the ages, figwort has been used for treating leg wounds. 'We think that it might be particularly promising for diabetes. Many of these patients suffer from leg ulcers which can, sadly, sometimes result in an amputation because there is not that much which works by way of treatment.'

Might the same discovery be made one day for a particular herbal remedy to treat an allergy such as hayfever? As the rise in allergies has continued, we've seen a worldwide increase in complementary treatments as people search for a more natural way to control their symptoms. Partly, this could be due to the fact that they may not like the idea of taking a conventional treatment such as steroids, and partly it could be because practitioners of complementary medicine are often able to give patients or their children more time to talk about their condition. This is why complementary therapies are often referred to as holistic medicine, because the practitioner tries to treat the 'whole person' rather than just focusing on their itchy skin or constricted lungs.

Go to Google and search under 'herbal remedies and allergy' and you will come up with thousands of websites, all selling you different remedies. The problem is, how can you tell what works? There is a distinct lack of scientific research in this field and, in fact, there are very few trials that actually show that herbal remedies have more success at treating the ailment than conventional medicine.

Just because it is a natural herb, doesn't mean that it can't harm you. Unfortunately, herbal remedies can have side effects in the same way that modern compounds can – the difference being that a tablet handed out by a family doctor will come with a leaflet telling you about the possible adverse reactions, whereas herbs will not. The other complication is that plants contain dozens of different substances, some of which may not suit you and may not suit the other medication you are taking. If you opt for a herbal remedy, you should always check first with your doctor or practitioner that it won't work negatively against your usual treatment.

Also, as Professor Simmonds at Kew Gardens has pointed out, plants of the same species can produce chemicals of very different potency, so it is important that scientists distinguish between the varieties. Another problem is that a freshly picked plant can act very differently from one that has dried out over a few days, as key components may decompose in that time.

While herbal remedies provide a whole range of compounds which are said to restore a holistic 'balance' to the body, Western pharmaceutical products are increasingly based on purified molecules that act on specific biological targets. But it isn't as simple as taking one extract from a plant and assuming that it can be transformed into an effective drug. The World Health Organisation (WHO), based in Geneva, have been investigating the application of herbal remedies. 'Purified compounds extracted from herbal remedies have a 90 per cent failure rate in clinical trials,' says Xiaorui Zhang, Coordinator of WHO's Traditional Medicine programme. 'So the synergistic effect between the different chemicals in a plant or plants has to be taken into consideration.'

WHO actively encourages research on the traditional use of herbal medicines, especially those that alleviate symptoms of diseases, such as malaria and AIDS. It has also developed guidelines for the clinical testing of traditional therapies and sponsors several centres worldwide that are compiling a database, in English, of information on natural medicines. The global market for herbal remedies is now thought to be around US$23 billion and growing, and many scientists think there is a bigger need to bridge the gap between traditional and Western-style medicine.

Can herbs help asthma?

Asthma has risen by more than 50 per cent in developed countries in the last twenty-five years (see Chapter Five). The extraordinary rate of increase has been accompanied by a quite natural desire to find complementary treatments which could offer another way of clearing the airways. Around two-thirds of those with mild asthma and around three-quarters of those with severe symptoms are believed to use herbal remedies to control the illness or relieve wheezing and breathlessness.

Unfortunately, there is a dearth of good knowledge and investigation into these potentially beneficial plants. When it comes to herbs that are said to contain chemicals to help with asthma, too little is known about any potential risks which may involve side effects. Or is it possible that some of these remedies, handed down in families over the years, work only as a placebo, making the patient feel better, psychologically, but not actually affecting the condition?

In 2000, Professor Edzard Ernst, one of Britain's leading scientific experts on alternative and complementary medicine, did a systematic review of all the trials that had been carried out to investigate the efficacy of herbal preparations on asthmatics. Six of the trials focused on traditional Chinese medicines, and eight on Indian Ayurvedic medicines. Three other trials looked at a Japanese Kampo medicine, marijuana, and dried ivy leaf extract. Analysis of the data showed that most of the trials were of poor quality and lacked the exacting criteria required for a thorough scientific appraisal. Among those that indicated some positive benefits, the flaws were such to cast doubt on the validity of the results.

Writing in the journal *Thorax*, in October 2000, Ernst said: 'There is no fully convincing evidence for any of the herbal preparations described.' He also warned that none of the herbal remedies referred to were likely to be free of side effects. Some even interfered with prescribed drugs. This is not simply a case of conventional scientists casting aspersions on anything alternative; what they would like to see, and have asked for, is a properly designed trial to assess the real safety and treatment value of herbal medicines for asthma. Yet, seven years on, there has still been no such trial – and I could find no evidence of one being planned.

Despite this being the case, many patients do resort to herbal remedies because they feel that symptoms can be alleviated. Often they hear of remedies by word of mouth, or through a herbalist, naturopath or other practitioners.

These are some of the traditional herbal remedies for asthma:

- **Camomile tea** is used as an antihistamine
- **Elderberry** relieves nasal congestion
- **Ginger** reduces allergic reaction
- **Green tea** opens bronchial passages
- **Hyssop tea** relieves respiratory congestion
- **Licorice root** increases mucus production to counter dry cough
- **Lobelia** tincture or capsules help reduce inflammatory reaction and soothe bronchial tissue
- **Mullein oil** relieves cough and helps clear bronchial tubes

Eczema

With this condition, there is some evidence that herbal remedies can help. Professor Ernst, who had found no evidence for herbs on asthma, did have more success when it came to eczema. In 1998, he looked at two trials where a herbal remedy was tested on some patients, with placebos (dummy medications) used on others. He concluded: 'There is preliminary evidence that Chinese herbs may be of benefit in the treatment of eczema in children and adults. Larger trials are required to adequately establish the benefit and harm of this treatment.'

Chinese herbalism is the most prevalent of the ancient herbal traditions currently practised in Britain. It is based on concepts of yin and yang and of Qi energy. Chinese herbs are ascribed qualities such as 'cooling' (yin) or 'stimulating' (yang) and used, often in combination, according to the deficiencies or excesses of these qualities in the patient.

Modern Western herbalism emphasises the effects of herbs on individual body systems. For example, herbs may be used for their supposed anti-inflammatory, haemostatic, expectorant, antispasmodic, or immunostimulatory properties. Herbs that have been traditionally used to treat eczema are listed below.

A naturopathic doctor or other herbal specialist might recommend one or more of these remedies after evaluating you and your eczema:

- **Burdock root** (*Arctium lappa*) – applied topically for skin inflammations
- **German camomile** (*Matricaria recutita*) – may reduce inflammation and speed wound healing
- **Goldenrod** (*Solidago virgaurea*) – applied topically for wound healing; has anti-inflammatory properties
- **Red clover** (*Trifolium pratense*) – has anti-inflammatory properties and has been used as an ointment for this skin condition
- **Stinging nettle** (*Urtica dioica*) – used down the centuries for helping childhood eczema. The nettle has a diuretic property and helps the body to expel uric acid. Herbalists suggest making it into a tea to drink regularly.

Lavender

Known mainly for its relaxing effects to aid with anxiety and insomnia, some herbalists recommend oral lavender for skin conditions such as eczema. In one study of topical lavender, however, children with eczema who received massage with or without lavender oil applied to the skin both did well. In other words, the improvement in the rash was related to the massage – whether lavender oil was used, or not, seemed to make no difference. To the extent that eczema is worsened by stress, it is possible that lavender adds some benefit by helping you relax.

154

Hayfever

It's no surprise that people with hayfever are keen to find out if there are herbs which contain compounds that might put an end to months of runny noses and watery eyes. Some people say that particular steam inhalations seem to make a difference, others swear by the herb eyebright.

Unfortunately, there is a lack of firm evidence that herbal remedies work any better than conventional drugs, with one exception – the herb butterbur, a perennial shrub found across Europe which, in the Middle Ages, was used to treat plague and fever. According to researchers who tested its properties in 2002, the extract of this plant appears to work as well as antihistamines, but does not have the side effect of drowsiness.

Hayfever sufferers should beware when drinking herbal teas because some of them may contain leaves or pollen grains which can actually trigger the allergy and make the symptoms worse. Doctors have warned that echinacea, a popular herbal remedy for colds in the UK, can trigger symptoms and anyone who knows they have a plant allergy should avoid this.

Beneficial herbs for hayfever include:

- **Eucalyptus** – used in steam inhalation to ease congestion
- **Eyebright** – tincture or capsules help reduce symptoms
- **Ginger** – reduces inflammation, antimicrobial
- **Licorice root** – reduces inflammation, antiviral, antibacterial
- **Nettle** – extract acts as an expectorant, reduces sinus inflammation

- **Rooibos** – has antihistamine properties. A tea is sometimes helpful in relieving symptoms

- **St John's Wort** – capsules are used to relieve sinus headache

Some herbs have the ability to do harm as well as good

Ephedra Known in Chinese as *Ma-huang*, ephedra is the plant whose active compound is used to make ephedrine, the drug which can save the life of a patient with a severe nut allergy or an asthma attack. But it is very powerful and it can also cause the body's blood vessels to go into contractions and narrow, resulting in death. Back in 2003, the US government decided to ban dietary supplements containing ephedra because of these concerns. At the time, around 15 million Americans were using the herb each year – usually in supplements to help them lose weight or raise their energy levels – but a series of studies led the regulatory body, the Food and Drug Administration, to decide that the risks were too high. There had already been an outcry over the death of a twenty-three-year-old baseball player, Steve Bechler, who fell ill after taking a supplement containing the herb.

Aristolochic acid This is a known cancer-causing chemical which can also do very severe kidney damage. In 2000, the Food and Drug Administration issued warnings about it following the kidney failures that had been seen across Europe. More than a hundred patients in Belgium were affected. One of the concerns is that this chemical is sometimes substituted for others in herbal preparations, making it hard for consumers to know what they are getting.

Ginkgo biloba This plant has been used medicinally for thousands of years and its leaves come from an ancient tree growing across China. It is a very common culinary ingredient in the Far East, as well as being one of the most popular medicinal herbs in the United States. Many different conditions are said to benefit from ginkgo and at the moment it is being investigated for its role in improving memory and concentration. Some say it can also help with coughs and asthma, as well as breathing difficulties. However, although it is generally safe, it should be used with great caution by patients who are on anti-coagulant therapy. The active compounds in the plant affect people's circulation and if you are taking other medications, talk to your doctor first before taking a supplement.

What to watch out for when you use complementary medicine

- The placebo effect. If you really want an complementary medical treatment to work, you may think it is working, even when it isn't. This can often be the case with complementary medicine and if you are also taking conventional medicine it is extremely difficult to know whether your symptoms are starting to improve because of this or because of the complementary medicine.

- Read the label. Every country requires labels to state how a herb or vitamin may affect the body, but they are not required to carry health warnings. Labels also cannot claim any medical or health benefit – although in the UK, there has been controversy over the government's decision to allow homeopathy remedies to make medical claims. Bear in mind that some products aren't properly labelled, particularly those imported from other countries. Many people experience toxic – sometimes deadly – effects from using improperly labelled herbs. Some products contain unnamed medicines such as steroids, anti-inflammatories or sedatives that act to reduce your symptoms. Other 'hidden ingredients' may be dangerous. Use only products that have been tested for safety and effectiveness – check with the manufacturer if the product doesn't tell you about the testing it has undergone.

- Follow directions. The Asthma and Allergy Foundation of America has warned patients not to increase the amount or frequency of a dose or use a treatment or device in a different way than recommended. Do not use herbs in combinations. Do not take herbs if you are pregnant or breastfeeding.

- Beware of developing allergy symptoms. Allergies to specific plants and other substances (such as nickel) can build up over time. Products you've used for years may suddenly cause mild to serious allergy symptoms, especially if you are already allergic to something else. Check if new herbs, foods or other products you plan to use are in the same 'family' as your known allergens.

- Consult your doctor before you begin a new treatment. It is essential that you tell your doctor about using complementary treatments, particularly if you have symptoms of asthma or allergy. The people in the health-food store or in the holistic clinic are helpful and know a lot about their subject, but they cannot make a diagnosis and they will not know enough about the conventional treatments.

Acupuncture

Karen Jones had her first asthma attack when she was twenty three and contracted a fungal infection in her lungs. Despite going on the appropriate medication, she found herself increasingly short of breath, particularly after she did any exercise. However, today, eight years on, she is almost symptom-free after only three months of acupuncture treatment. 'I wish I had found out about acupuncture earlier,' she says. 'A friend recommended it after hearing it mentioned on a radio programme. I don't quite understand why it works but all I know is that it does really do it for me.'

The use of acupuncture for asthma is not new – in fact, it is one of the oldest and most widespread complementary techniques. The first documented history of acupuncture is ascribed to the legendary Yellow Emperor (Huang Di) in China, around 2000 BC. In the second part of his classic book, he describes his desire to relieve the suffering of his subjects afflicted with disease, shunning the poisons of medicine in favour of fine needles to harmonise the blood and Qi energy.

Unlike some other complementary therapies, there is a body of evidence to recommend acupuncture. In 1996, at the request of the US Food and Drug Administration, Dr Kim Jobst reviewed studies on the effectiveness of acupuncture for asthma. Dr Jobst, an experienced acupuncturist and research fellow in the department of pharmacology at Oxford University in the UK, reviewed sixteen published studies and concluded that acupuncture was proven effective in ten of them. Of a total of 320 patients in the studies, 91 per cent who used acupuncture were able to reduce the amount of medication they required. 'Patients should not stop taking their asthma medication but there is evidence that acupuncture can be effective in reducing the severity of the disease and the amount of medication – which can cause severe side effects – that a patient needs,' concluded Dr Jobst.

Relaxation techniques

Living with a chronic condition such as an allergy can be really stressful and one point which everyone can agree on is that relieving this tension has to be a primary aim. There are several different relaxation techniques, which have been used down the ages to deal with a range of illnesses, and some of these seem to be particularly useful for patients who are hypersensitive. The techniques have their roots in spiritual beliefs, but people of any, or no, religion can use these methods to help ease their condition.

• What stress does to you

Your emotional and physical reactions to stress are partly determined by the sensitivity of your sympathetic nervous system. You may have heard of the 'fight or flight' reaction that people have when they are stressed or excited, which leads to a racing pulse, changes in breathing, muscle tension and even affects the circulation.

158

If you have an especially stressful life, your sympathetic nervous system may always be poised to react to a crisis, putting you in a state of constant tension. In this mode, you tend to react to small stresses the same way you would react to real emergencies. Repeated episodes of the fight or flight reaction deplete your energy reserves and, if they continue, cause a downward spiral that can lead to emotional burnout and eventually complete exhaustion. You can break this spiral only by learning to manage stress in a way that protects and even increases your energy level. This is what many relaxation programmes aim to do – but different kinds suit different people. Many find yoga very therapeutic, but not everyone takes to it.

These are some of the techniques used by the Cleveland Clinic in Ohio, USA, reprinted with their kind permission.

- **Rhythmic breathing** If your breathing is short and hurried, slow it down by taking long, slow breaths. Inhale slowly, then exhale slowly. Count slowly to five as you inhale and then count slowly to five as you exhale. As you exhale slowly, pay attention to how your body naturally relaxes. Recognising this change will help you to relax even more.

- **Deep breathing** Imagine a spot just below your navel. Breathe into that spot, filling your abdomen with air. Let the air fill you from the abdomen up, then let it out, like deflating a balloon. With every long, slow exhalation, you should feel more relaxed.

- **Visualised breathing** Find a comfortable place where you can close your eyes and combine slowed breathing with your imagination. Picture relaxation entering your body and tension leaving your body. Breathe deeply but in a natural rhythm. Visualise your breath coming into your nostrils, going into your lungs and expanding your chest and abdomen. Then, visualise your breath going out the same way. Continue breathing, but each time you inhale, imagine that you are breathing in more relaxation. Each time you exhale, imagine that you are getting rid of a little more tension.

- **Progressive muscle relaxation** Switch your thoughts to yourself and your breathing. Take a few deep breaths, exhaling slowly. Mentally scan your body. Notice areas that feel tense or cramped. Quickly loosen up these areas. Let go of as much tension as you can. Rotate your head in a smooth, circular motion once or twice. (Stop any movements that cause pain!) Roll your shoulders forwards and backwards several times. Let all of your muscles completely relax. Recall a pleasant thought for a few seconds. Take another deep breath and exhale slowly. You should feel relaxed.

159

- **Relax to music** Combine relaxation exercises with your favourite music in the background. Select the type of music that lifts your mood or that you find soothing or calming. Some people find it easier to relax while listening to specially designed relaxation tapes, which provide music and relaxation instructions.

- **Mental imagery relaxation** Mental imagery relaxation, or guided imagery, is a proven form of focused relaxation that helps create harmony between the mind and body. Guided imagery coaches you in creating calm, peaceful images in your mind – a 'mental escape'. Identify your self-talk, that is, what you are saying to yourself about what is going on with your illness. It is important to identify negative self-talk and develop healthy, positive self-talk. By making affirmations, you can counteract negative thoughts and emotions.

• Yoga

This practice, or philosophy, has been used by many people with illness in order to lead a healthier life and to attain a focus and a calm outlook which will help them deal with their condition. It can be successful in so many ways and, for people who have allergies, the focus on breathing exercises and meditation is particularly welcome. Before you join a class, make sure your instructor is aware of any medical conditions you might have, especially asthma, as it does involve learning new breathing exercises.

• Aromatherapy

This very popular form of therapy involves massaging different blended essential oils into the body to produce a sense of well-being. Those with allergies should be very aware of the fact that some of these oils may be harmful and trigger a reaction. There is also the danger that the oils can irritate the skin of those who have eczema. These risks are small, as long as the oils are used properly. Remember that essential oils must always be diluted in a suitable carrier oil, and should never be drunk or swallowed. The ones that can often cause a sensitivity reaction include cinnamon, sage, clove and hyssop. Make sure you are seen by a qualified therapist who should, as a matter of course, ask you about any allergies at the beginning of the consultation.

• Hypnotherapy

Despite all the ridiculous claims made on websites, it is simply not possible to cure an allergy with hypnosis. There are hypnotherapists who say that in the atopic person, the brain is 'making a mistake' when it comes into contact with an allergen like pollen. That kind of misunderstanding can be dangerous because it misleads people who may not have learned about the real nature of allergies. However, hypnotherapy in its correct form can be used to help alleviate stress or any feelings of anxiety that are exacerbating the allergy, and so, indirectly, it can help the patient. Always ensure that you see a registered hypnotherapist, and, again, do make sure you tell your doctor in case there are any problems later on.

• Breathe easy

Breathing can play an extremely important part in helping someone deal with symptoms and improve their health. We all take it for granted that we breathe in the right way, but when your lungs are not functioning properly it's very easy to get into bad habits. The most common problem is hyperventilation, where people start to take too much air in, or 'over-breathe'. If this carries on for some time, it can leave you with a strange set of symptoms, which include an aching chest, dizziness, an abnormal heart rhythm and a pins and needles sensation in the hands and feet.

When we breathe, the oxygen in the air is taken into the lungs and absorbed into the bloodstream via the tiny capillaries which are threaded across the lung surface. As the oxygen enters the capillaries, carbon dioxide leaves them, and this goes into the lungs and is exhaled as you breathe out. This exchange of gases is very important because the levels of carbon dioxide in the blood affect many different organs. If you hyperventilate, the levels of carbon dioxide in the blood start to go up and down a great deal and this in turn affects the nerves.

Anyone can hyperventilate, and this is what happens when someone suffers a panic attack, but it is especially common in people with asthma, which is why it is so important that they are aware of it. Doctors can help patients to see if they are hyperventilating with some simple tests and also by asking about their symptoms. There are a series of special exercises that can be done to correct any problems.

• The Buteyko method

This technique is growing in popularity, as it has been shown to be safe for treating asthma patients. Several trials have proved that it can reduce the symptoms and some work has also suggested that it may reduce the need of reliever medication for asthmatics, although this is a controversial claim. The method is part of a health philosophy pioneered by the Russian doctor Konstantin Buteyko, who believed that asthma was actually caused by hyperventilation. This is not true, but there is little doubt now that the technique can help many patients.

The way in which these exercises work is that they correct abnormal breathing patterns. They help to unblock the nose and train the patient to breathe through the nose rather than the mouth. The technique is aimed at increasing the patient's 'control pause' – the amount of time the individual can spend between breaths. This does not involve holding your breath, but pausing between an exhalation and then an inhalation.

Proponents of the method say that by using reduced breathing exercises, people are able to increase their control pause up to several minutes and thus decrease their symptoms. Breathing through the nose, rather than the mouth, is also important. This can protect the airways, since the air is cleaned and warmed when it goes through the nose, and reduces the desire to hyperventilate.

If you are interested in this method, you can find a local class in your area, or you can do the exercises at home by buying a book on the method or using a video or DVD to instruct yourself on the technique. Again, it's a good idea to chat it through with your doctor.

The most important thing is not to stop taking your regular medication even if you are using these methods. Some practitioners claim that the technique means you no longer need medication, but this is an untested theory – and potentially a dangerous one if damage is being done to the lungs when you come off medication.

162

A nurse with a mission

One woman who has put all of her faith – and a lot of her money – into the Buteyko Method is nurse Jill McGowan. The forty-five-year-old Scot, who has won several awards for her work, became convinced that the treatment could make a huge difference to asthma sufferers.

Back in 1996, she learned the method for herself and found that it completely alleviated her own asthma symptoms. She then trained to become a Buteyko practitioner and set up the Buteyko Institute Trust, raising £55,000 by selling her own home and donating three-quarters of her £30,000 annual salary for two years. A pilot study, which she pushed through in 2003, resulted in a 96 per cent success rate in relieving symptoms. Jill now runs regular courses in hospitals and health centres across the United Kingdom and Ireland for individuals suffering not just from asthma, but also chronic bronchitis, emphysema, sleep apnoea, snoring, allergies, rhinitis, sinusitis, and multiple sclerosis – to name but a few conditions.

Jill, who is also a lecturer in nursing at Paisley University, near Glasgow, Scotland says, 'I knew I wasn't going to get backing from pharmaceutical companies but I wanted others to benefit. To get Buteyko accepted by the NHS, it needs to be tested under proper conditions.'

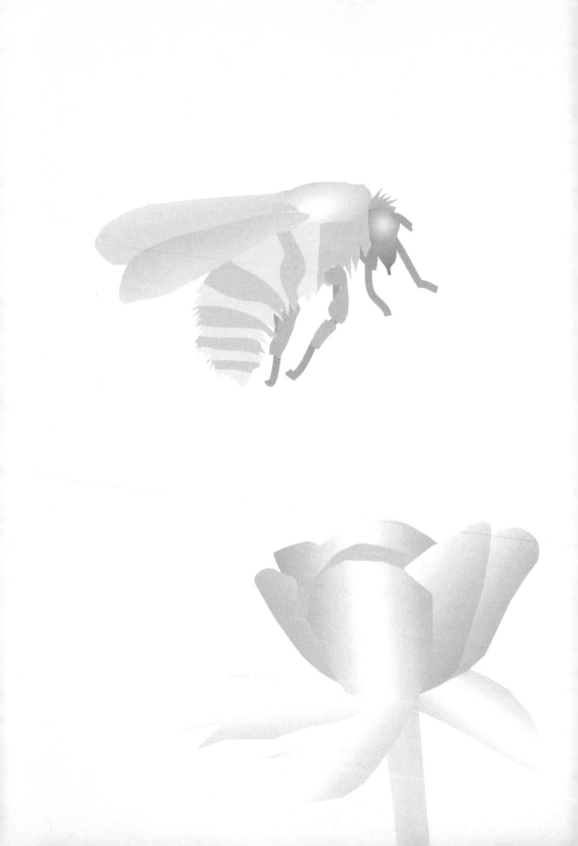

CHAPTER TWELVE
YOUR HOME

If you could see a house-dust mite under a microscope, it would remind you of some monster created by the special effects team of a horror movie. It has pincers and a scaly, armoured back, and moves very slowly. These tiny bugs (proper name *Dermatophagoides pteronyssinus*), smaller than a full stop on this page, have been around for millennia. It has been calculated that they have been in existence for 23 million years – but only started to co-exist with man 10,000 years ago. How they even survive is quite astonishing. They are blind, cannot drink or take in food and survive by absorbing moisture and oxygen from the atmosphere.

Perhaps most astonishingly of all, the mite uses its droppings as 'food parcels'. There are strong enzymes contained within the excrement that are able to break down hard-to-digest food for later nourishment. These enzymes cause and trigger allergies in humans, as they attack the delicate living tissue that is actually a human's respiratory passage. As the house-dust mite lives inside mattresses, pillows, upholstery, cushions and soft toys, the allergens, which affect millions of people with asthma, are sprayed out into the air every time you get into bed, turn over at night or sit down on a sofa or armchair.

It is not the dust itself that is harmful, but the presence of the mites. If the air is dry, the creatures will not be able to survive. Getting rid of these creatures is not easy. The mite can produce up to twenty droppings a day, which means approximately 2,000 during its active lifetime of up to three to four months. The adult female can lay up to a hundred eggs depending upon living conditions, which need to be warm, dark and damp.

There is one chink of weakness, however, the house-dust mite's biological make-up is 75 per cent water. So, to continue to breed, they have to live in a moist atmosphere. Reducing moisture in the home is a threat to their existence. When the humidity falls below 50 per cent, the mites gradually dry out and are killed.

 Are you safe in your bed?

You might think of it as a place of rest and relaxation but, in fact, your bed is also a prime habitat for a huge amount of 'invisible' life. It's not a very nice thought, but a typical used mattress can have anything between 100,000 to 10 million mites inside. (10 per cent of the weight of a two-year-old pillow can be composed of dead mites and their droppings.) This is because they like warm, moist surroundings such as the inside of a mattress when someone is on it. Humans shed about one-fifth of an ounce of dander (dead skin) each week and this is what the mites like to eat.

The use of chemicals

There are a whole range of products on sale that promise to kill off house-dust mites – sprays, air fresheners, carpet shampoos and air filtration systems. Unfortunately, there is very little independent evidence out there to show whether or not they work. Sufferers should bear in mind that not only can they be quite expensive, but also that constantly spraying different rooms is very time-consuming.

These products are not necessarily useless, but the proper research has failed to show any benefit to symptoms or any other worthwhile aspect of asthma. There are chemicals which do kill mites, but it may be the case that it is impossible to use them in sufficient doses in a normal house for them to be really effective.

The other unanswered worry is about the toxicity of these chemicals, given that children and adults will be exposed to them. It's easy to spend an awful lot of money in the war against these bugs, but sometimes the simplest of methods can be just as effective. For asthmatics, any measure which keeps dust mites at bay is helpful because they are one of the biggest triggers of asthma attack. A big review carried out in 1998 has suggested that many of the strategies aimed at minimising sufferers' exposure to the mites, either by killing the bugs, or by sealing them off from human contact, do not seem very effective. Researchers from Denmark, Sweden and Wales have found that no technique has helped to reduce symptoms in asthmatics effectively. The scientists, writing in the *British Medical Journal*, looked at the outcome of twenty-three separate studies that tested the impact of both chemical and physical methods to reduce exposure to mites. The BMJ trial looked at all randomised trials worldwide that compared chemical (also known as acaricidal) or physical measures, such as vacuum cleaning, heating, barrier methods using special bedding sheets or air filtration systems to control mites.

But the BMJ study found that forty one out of 113 patients who tested the treatments showed an improvement in their condition. However, thirty eight out of 117 asthma sufferers who tested no treatment also registered an improvement in symptoms. The researchers concluded that the treatments had no significant impact.

Dr Michael Burr, a consultant in public health medicine at the University of Wales, said new methods were needed to tackle the problem. He also said that existing treatments needed to be better targeted at people who were most likely to benefit. 'It is of very little value to just give blanket instructions to everybody with mite-sensitive asthma to do lots of rather tedious things which will not do them very much good.

'There may be many factors causing the asthma, including allergy to cats and cigarette smoke. We need to identify those people who will really benefit from addressing the dust-mite problem.'

Dr Burr said methods which simply killed the mites were useless because the droppings remained behind. It was also important not to concentrate treatment on one possible site, such as a bed mattress, when the mites may have infested many other areas.

A possible vaccine?

One scientific objective is to create a vaccine against dust-mite allergy. Cytos, a Swiss vaccine company, carried out a small study of their dust-mite vaccine, which has revealed promising results in 2006. Patients given the vaccine – which uses DNA material – experienced far fewer allergy symptoms such as sneezing, while asthmatics did not experience any attacks. The Cytos vaccine uses one particular protein from the dust-mite excrement – the allergen – which would usually cause an allergic reaction. It is designed to boost the activity of the immune system to suppress that allergic reaction.

Of nineteen patients injected in a Cytos study to check the safety and efficacy of its vaccine, seventeen were found to be completely tolerant to the mites, having no allergic reactions. But it is still early days, and trials need to be carried out on thousands more patients before the vaccine could become available.

Aside from the plague of house-dust mites which can obviously cause such misery for those with specific allergies, there are other areas within the home that can also cause allergy sufferers big problems.

Carpets and furnishings

We all need furnishings and flooring but, for some of us, even the surroundings we choose for our homes can prompt an allergic response. Furniture, flooring and shelving that is made from chipboard or MDF (medium-density fibreboard) may trigger asthma symptoms. This is because it contains formaldehyde resin, which gives off a pungent, colourless gas that can irritate the airways.

Carpets are not only a breeding ground for house-dust mites, but they also give off this gas and reported symptoms include upper respiratory irritations, headaches, skin rashes, shortness of breath, cough and fatigue. If you're buying a new carpet, always ask the shop to unroll it and allow it to air before it is laid down in your home.

Many carpets come with a foam underlay which can also be a problem by triggering a response in those who are allergic to latex. There are different types of underlay available; always check with your retailer before you buy.

Whenever you walk into a soft furnishing department, you can smell the chemicals given off by new sofas and chairs. The store you go to should be able to air the furniture for you for a week or so before it is brought into the house. Once it arrives, try to keep the windows open and the house aired for a few days.

According to the National Institute of Environmental Health Studies in America, the distinct odour of new carpet is usually due to the chemical known as 4-phenylcyclohexene (4-PC). This chemical can be detected at very low levels, but does not result in an unpleasant smell for everyone and usually goes within a few days.

One possible solution for people who are sensitive to these chemicals is to go for natural wooden floors rather than carpets, and venetian blinds, which can be wiped down easily, rather than curtains. If you are worried about the sofa, you could opt for wooden or bamboo chairs with loose cushions fitted on top which can be easily washed or fitted with special covers.

Dampness

Houses that suffer from damp have been linked with asthma in some people because mould spores can trigger an allergic response. Research has also shown that, during the winter months, asthma symptoms are harder to control in people who live in homes without central heating. There is no one type of heating that is best for all allergy sufferers, but there does seem to be a link between poor housing conditions and allergies.

Wood and coal fires

Wood and coal fires which don't have proper flues to take away the smoke can cause mild worsening of breathing problems. However, if the flues are working properly, these type of fires can be more suitable for those who suffer with asthma as they are less house-dust-mite friendly.

Gas stoves can be a problem because they produce nitrogen dioxide, a gas which can harm the airways. There is some evidence to suggest that if a child inhales the gas and also lives in a house with cats and dogs, the combination of the different allergens makes them far more likely to develop asthma. An efficient extractor fan in a cooker hood can take away some of the gas given off by a hob.

Good ventilation is important and having a house that is draughty may help alleviate allergic conditions since it makes it harder for the pollutants to settle.

Cleaning

A wide assortment of domestic products and solvents are used around the home, many of which release chemicals that can cause breathing difficulties in some people who have asthma. These chemicals are known as volatile organic compounds (VOCs). Many household and DIY products such as cleaning fluids, varnishes, glue, paints, furniture polish, air fresheners, carpet cleaners, oven cleaners and dry-cleaned clothes all contain VOCs.

The US regulator, the Environment Protection Agency (EPA), carried out a Total Exposure Assessment Methodology (TEAM) and found levels of around a dozen common VOC pollutants to be two to five times higher inside homes rather than outside, regardless of whether the homes were located in rural or highly industrial areas. Additional TEAM studies indicate that while people are using products containing VOCs, they can expose themselves and others to very high pollutant levels and elevated concentrations can persist in the air long after the activity is completed.

The EPA, the agency tasked by the US government with protecting human health and the environment, monitors environmental pollutants. On its website, it warns: 'Key signs or symptoms associated with exposure to VOCs include conjunctival irritation, nose and throat discomfort, headache, allergic skin reaction, dyspnea, declines in serum cholinesterase levels, nausea, emesis, epistaxis, fatigue and dizziness.'

It also explains that, at present, not much is known about what health effects occur from the levels of VOCs usually found in homes: 'Many VOC compounds are known to cause cancer in animals; some are suspected of causing, or are known to cause, cancer in humans.'

It's obviously going to be hard to avoid these chemicals completely, but one answer may be to use solid or liquid alternatives that aren't released into the air, instead of sprays. The other important factor is to use as little of the product as possible and then open windows. If it causes you a real problem, ask someone else to do the cleaning and stay out of the room for a few hours.

Another suggestion is to wear a face mask covering your nose and mouth, while doing the cleaning but, unfortunately, there isn't a lot of research to show that they reduce symptoms although, anecdotally, some patients do say they make a real difference.

Beware of research found in sales literature that claim that their products are successful at achieving specific results (e.g. removing allergens) – these will have often been conducted by the manufacturer. Although it can be shown that a product can remove an allergen, this is not the same as showing that it reduces the frequency of symptoms in a person using it.

• Vacuum cleaners

Hoovering with ordinary vacuum cleaners can present problems because they throw up all the dust – and the bits of mite – into the air. Tiny parts of the faeces then fly across a room, spreading the allergen even further.

There is now a large industry built around vacuum cleaners that have anti-allergy filters. Many of them have what is known as a HEPA (high efficiency particulate air) filter which claim to extract far more dust and far more fine particles. One of the problems, however, can be that the dust can escape through the different joints of a cleaner, particularly as they age.

Like many other anti-allergy devices, it is hard to know what really works because each machine is tested by the manufacturer, with very little independent evaluation. Investing in an expensive vacuum cleaner with anti-allergy filters may not always be a wise buy.

So how do you know whether your vacuum cleaner works? Many people turn to the consumer magazine *Which?* for product reviews and in April 2007 the magazine testing twenty four different cleaners made by thirteen different brands, all commonly available in the leading retailer. It found that cylinder cleaners emerged as much better at retaining allergen particles, particularly cat and dog hair. Makers Miele, which specialise in cylinders, came out of top and the magazine's Best Buy was their Cat & Dog TT 5000 make. It found that the filter was better at retaining the pet hairs than other makes, but the magazine did not look at whether finer particles are likely to escape through other parts of the cylinder.

If you are thinking of buying a new vacuum cleaner, you could ask the manufacturer how much allergen remains in the air after vacuuming a room – this is the best test of whether it works. There is a cleaner known as a Medivac that is a whole unit which is installed in the house with pipes going into different rooms. A hose can then be attached to each wall pipe and the room cleaned. Tests have shown that it does remove mite faeces, however, it is a big expense and a major installation project.

As this book was going to press, it was revealed that a new kind of vacuum cleaner, which uses dust compression technology, was being launched in the UK in 2007. The LG Compressor, made by a South Korean company, claims to suck up three times as much dirt as most rivals and then compresses it into solid blocks which are easier to throw away. One model is specifically anti-allergic with different levels of filter to take out all the particulates.

This news will be a relief for those who suffer from asthma or other allergies that are made worse by the tiny airborne particles in household dust, however, somewhat alarmingly, research suggests that more than half of all adults in Britain only vacuum once a month or more – far less often than had been thought.

Decorating

There has been little medical research on the many chemicals used in renovating or decorating a home. Wet paint can cause problems as it gives off chemicals that can trigger asthma symptoms in some people. If you have noticed such adverse effects, look out for the new low-odour, water-based gloss paints that should be available from any large DIY store.

Stripping wallpaper can unsettle dust, so wash down wallpaper before starting to help to dampen down the dust. Ensure there is plenty of ventilation. Again, while wearing a mask can be helpful while performing this task.

How to win the war against indoor allergens

- Ventilation
  - Good ventilation benefits people with asthma. It reduces humidity, which reduces the number of house-dust mites and moulds. It also helps to disperse gases produced by heating and cooking.
  - Opening the window generates a significant amount of air exchange.
  - Free-standing fans or extractor fans that are placed so that they aid air flow to and from the outside environment, without blowing allergens around within the room, may help.

- Air conditioning and ventilation in buildings with no windows is more controversial. Some researchers suggest that they merely re-circulate allergens and mould spores, especially if the rooms are not properly ventilated.

• Ionisers

These are devices which use a high voltage to ionise, or electrically charge, molecules of air. The idea behind them is that in a natural outdoor environment, there is a balance between positive and negative ions – the charges contained in each. But in enclosed indoor space, the negative ions are depleted. The positively charged air attracts and holds suspended dust particles, which can cause fatigue, headaches, allergies and irritation of the eyes and mucous membranes. Ionisers claim to restore the electrical balance by neutralising the positive ions – the dust particles fall and are attracted to the ioniser. Although there is some evidence to suggest that ionisers can reduce allergens, other research shows that they can also increase symptoms, such as night-time coughs in children, and many scientists do not recommend their use.

• Air filters

HEPA filters are said to remove at least 99.97 per cent of the smallest airborne particles. They are made from mats that have fibres arranged to trap the very small particles that would normally escape. But although they pass the laboratory test and should, in theory, help people with allergies, there is still a lack of good data to show what they achieve when it comes to reducing symptoms.

Several studies have shown that modern air filters can capture allergens, but evidence that they are capable of reducing symptoms is less clear. The charity, Asthma UK, says that on the basis of the current science, they cannot recommend them until there is clearer evidence that they do work. The filters do appear to be effective for some, but only if other measures to control allergens are used alongside them, such as getting rid of the carpets in a house. If you are considering buying an air filter, find out what kind of allergens they capture. Some, such as cat dander, are so tiny that they can pass through most filters.

Tips for having a cleaner, less allergenic environment

- Have as little soft furniture as possible where house-dust mites may thrive.

- Use a wet cloth to clean walls, woodwork and floors. The floor can be polished.

- Wash your bedding regularly at a temperature of at least 60 degrees centigrade and buy cotton sheets, washable bottom sheets and synthetic blankets or duvets. Woollen blankets or quilts should be dry-cleaned. When bedding has been washed, hang it on the line if you can to keep it free of mites.

- Don't be tempted to dry your clothes in your bedroom or any other room because it adds to the moisture. House-dust mites can also live in clothes. If you have lots of woolly sweaters or jackets, have them regularly dry-cleaned – although this can be expensive, the dry-cleaning process will kill mites.

- Use wet cloths and a vacuum cleaner with a no-bag vortex and allergen filter to clean the house thoroughly, preferably every day, but at least twice a week.

- Avoid dust traps such as teddy bears, cushions, dried flowers, bric-a-brac and soft toys.

- Put duvets and pillows in plastic bags and put them in the freezer for 24 hours at least once a month to kill the mites.

- Try to air the house every day and don't use an air humidifier, which will only make matters worse. If the lower edge of the window is moist when you wake up in the morning, there is too much humidity in the air.

- Avoid the use of spray air fresheners, cleaners and so on because they may worsen your symptoms.

- Don't allow smoking in the house. If guests want to smoke, ask them to step outside!

The great outdoors?

• Pollution

Being outside on a lovely summer's day can trigger a host of allergic reactions, unfair as that seems. One pollutant that people have become particularly aware of in recent years is ozone, a chemical that is produced when car exhaust fumes hit sunlight, producing a highly reactive form of oxygen. The UK now gives out warnings when the ozone levels are high (levels tend to peak in the late afternoon and early evening), because for some people with asthma the effects can be devastating – serious enough to warrant hospitalisation.

This chemical affects the mucous membranes, especially the respiratory tract. When ozone reaches the cells, it can make breathing difficult and produces coughing, wheezing and shortness of breath. It also increases the vulnerability of the lungs to infection. Those particularly susceptible include young children, the elderly as well as people with asthma, chronic bronchitis or emphysema. However, scientists have come to realise that even healthy adults may experience such symptoms if a lot of time is spent outdoors or vigorous exercise is carried out during periods of high ozone levels.

Other air pollutants such as sulphur dioxide produced by heavy industry can also exacerbate the effect of ozone.

According to Dr David Peden, a professor of paediatrics at the University of North Carolina School of Medicine, USA, there can be a delayed reaction to the ozone levels. He and his colleagues looked at the effects of ozone on people allergic to dust mites. Not only did ozone worsen allergy symptoms immediately, but among patients with asthma, researchers found there was a chronic inflammation of the airways that could be measured the next day.

This is probably why people often end up being admitted to hospital one or two days after a high ozone day. 'There seems to be a time lag between the start of the inflammation and the effects that bring people to the emergency room,' says Peden.

Other research has shown that the tiny particles in diesel exhaust can increase a person's sensitivity to pollen or dust mites or other allergy-producing antigens. One way to cut down on exposure to ozone is to exercise outdoors in the morning, rather than the afternoon when the ozone levels peak at around 4pm. If you have to spend a lot of time in the car in heavy traffic, make sure you have air conditioning, which will cut down on the number of diesel particles coming into the car while you drive. These are known as particulates and are a mixture of soot and other chemicals which get into the nose and airways.

• Insect stings

Nearly everyone has been stung by an insect at one time or another. It's not a pleasant sensation and not one you would wish to repeat but, for most people, it's a matter of a short, sharp pain and a little red swelling that goes down quite quickly. However, for some – around one or two in every thousand – a sting is much more dangerous, because they suffer an allergic reaction to the venom contained in it.

Stinging insects all come from the group known as *Hymenoptera*, which includes wasps, bees and ants. The stinger itself – the sword-like bit that goes into your skin – was once used for egg laying, so only female insects can sting.

There is some evidence that the number of people suffering insect stings, and also a severe reaction from them, is on the rise. This is linked to climate change, since milder winters enable the insects to survive for longer and create more colonies in the spring. Worldwide, there are more than 100,000 different known wasp species. The term 'wasp' is generally associated with the yellowjackets *Vespula vulgaris* and *Vespula germanica*, which are the most troublesome group of social wasps for humans.

An interesting study, carried out by doctors at the Charite (Charity) Hospital in Berlin, Germany, between 2002 to 2004, looked at all the patients who came in with wasp sting injuries and evaluated the frequency, localisation, treatment (such as an adrenaline shot) as well as occurrence of allergic reactions and other complications. Researchers found that in this two-year period, the number of patients with insect stings had tripled. Alarmingly, the severity level increased as well due to the sharp increase in the number of internal stings after people had accidentally swallowed or breathed in a wasp.

They concluded that what they were seeing was a climate-related increase in the number of sting injuries. In Germany, 2003 had been a 'record' summer for its heat and the mild winter that followed meant the survival of lots of queen wasps who then created many new wasp colonies in 2004.

Britain has also seen an increase in serious stings. A total of 842 people were admitted for medical care following insect stings between April 2004 to March 2005 compared to 369 in the previous year. Experts say the sudden rise could be due to a new invasive species of aggressive wasp which has arrived in the

UK from the Continent. Professor Lars Chittka, an expert in Behavioural Ecology at Queen Mary College, University of London, told the BBC that Britain had seen an increase in the numbers of this newcomer wasp, called *Dolichovespula media*, in recent years. He described the new species as 'reasonably aggressive, who build relatively small nests in trees and bushes at eye height'.

Most stings occur at the end of summer, when people are out and about and the wasp colonies are at their peak size. At this time of year, the wasps can't find as many natural food sources and turn to ice creams and food left outside, increasing their contact with people.

- In Britain, wasp stings are far more common than bee stings and so too are the numbers who are allergic to them. On average, four or five bee or wasp stings cause a fatal anaphylactic shock (see page 178) in the UK every year. This isn't a huge number by any means, but for those who know they are allergic to the venom, going outside in the summer can be a nightmare.

- In the US, the Fire Ant can cause allergy and anaphylaxis.

- The Australian 'Jack Jumper Ant' (*Myrmecia pilosula*) is a medium-sized black bull ant prevalent down the eastern side of Australia and Tasmania. It is a very aggressive ant and its stings cause severe local pain. Severe allergic reactions are much more common than is seen with more common bull ants. Native Australian bees and the Green Ant of Queensland can also cause allergic reactions.

• What happens when you are stung

Stingers are very effective weapons because they deliver venom that causes pain when it pierces your skin. The major pain-causing chemical in a honey bee sting is melittin and it works by stimulating the nerve endings of pain receptors in the skin. The result is a very painful sensation, which begins as a sharp pain that lasts a few minutes and then becomes a dull ache.

A normal reaction is for the body to move fluid from the blood to the sting site, which causes the redness and swelling that is seen quite quickly. The swelling is likely to be bigger if you've been stung recently by the same kind of insect and it's also likely to be quite itchy.

Oral and topical antihistamines help prevent or reduce the itching and swelling. Try not to rub or scratch the sting site because microbes from the surface of the skin could be introduced into the wound and result in an infection.

Some people actually develop an allergy to the venom. In a wasp, it's an enzyme known as Antigen 5; in a bee, the enzyme which is producing this hypersensitive reaction is phospholipase.

178

You can become allergic after a single sting, or after many. Skin-prick tests are generally accurate for the diagnosis of insect venom allergy, but do carry a small risk of inducing a severe allergic reaction since traces of the venom are applied to the skin during testing. Around 10 per cent of patients who experience wasp anaphylaxis will have negative allergy tests because the tests aren't always completely accurate.

• Anaphylaxis

In allergic persons, the different parts of the venom circulating in the body combine with antibodies that are associated with mast cells (see pages 27–41) which are lying on vital organs. The mast cells release histamine and other biologically active substances, but this results in a leakage of fluid out of the blood and into the body tissues.

Reactions suffered range from mild – with redness and swelling, intense itching and pain all occurring within minutes of the sting – to a severe reaction which would include great itching, faintness, sweating, a pounding headache, stomach cramps and vomiting, as well as a choking sensation as the throat swells up. This happens when the person goes into anaphylactic shock – blood pressure drops dangerously low and fluid builds up in the lungs. If this response is not reversed within a short time, the patient could die.

Luckily, it can be reversed these days with fast, emergency treatment such as a shot of epinephrine (adrenaline) injected into the body. Individuals who are aware that they are allergic to stings should carry epinephrine in either a normal syringe (sting kit) or an auto-injector (EpiPen) whenever they think they might encounter stinging insects. (See page 120 for advice on how to use an EpiPen). Prompt action is imperative in this situation, since an allergic person can collapse within ten minutes of being stung.

Researchers have found that people who go into anaphylactic shock tend to have permanently raised concentrations of an enzyme called tryptase in their blood. They believe it could be possible to test people who develop an allergic reaction for levels of this enzyme after being stung.

Researchers from Ludwig-Maximilians University at Munich, Germany, carried out tests on patients who were allergic to bee and wasp stings. They carried out blood tests at least two weeks after they had been stung. The tests revealed that nine out of twelve (75 per cent) patients with high levels of tryptase in their blood suffered severe reactions. However, only twenty eight of the 102 (28 per cent) patients with lower tryptase concentrations experienced the same severity of reaction.

• Avoiding stings

Bees and wasps can be attracted to the perfumes found naturally within a garden and the same applies to the scent you may be wearing. It's a good idea not to use a perfume or wash with a scented soap if you're going out into an area where there may be bees or wasps. Avoid going barefoot on grass, especially areas where there is clover or other perfumed ground flowers, and don't wear brightly coloured or patterned clothing which will also attract these insects.

Rather than swipe furiously at bees and wasps when they come near you, it is better to remain calm, even if one lands on your skin, and wait for them to leave of their own accord. If you cannot wait for them to fly off, gently and slowly brush the insect away with a piece of paper. When swimming in pools, watch out for bees or wasps trapped on the surface of the water. It is always best to remove them to avoid being stung.

CHAPTER THIRTEEN
SUMMARY

What is it that people most fear in life? For some, it would be a violent, unprovoked attack, loss of their home, the death of a child or a diagnosis of cancer. Allergies are generally not something that people perceive as an immediate and deadly threat because, thankfully, for the majority of people they can be controlled and treated with a combination of the right medical advice, the right therapies and some lifestyle changes.

But no one, least of all national policymakers, should be under any doubt as to the huge impact they can have on someone's life. A woman with eczema can find it very hard to go out and socialise, hard to hold down a job, hard to find a partner. Equally, the child with a peanut allergy will be the child who cannot go to the birthday party for fear that a nut component may have been used in the food somewhere. Every time they go to a friend, their parent will have to tell the other parents how to use an EpiPen in case they suddenly go into anaphylatic shock. School trips can be tricky. As for eating out in a restaurant, that becomes a no-no for many families.

Allergies are a modern illness. They barely existed a hundred years ago, and now they affect nearly one in three of us. The reasons for why we have seen such a surge in conditions such as hayfever are complex, but need to be understood. In 1932, just one in thirty people suffered from a hypersensitivity – how could that rate have gone up tenfold in just three generations?

Some experts have argued that allergy is an index of cultural anxiety, showing how concerned we are about our lives, our environment and our cleanliness. But the illnesses that I have described in this book are real, not the figment of imagination, and can cause real pain and distress. It is becoming clearer, however, that to a large extent the path we have taken towards an ever-more hygienic world has created this conundrum, and that perhaps we need to look again at our obsession with defeating bacteria.

The most widely accepted theory to explain the allergy increase is that in Western nations the developing immune systems of babies are exposed to fewer challenges, largely because of the widespread use of antibiotics, more varied forms of food and water, and better living conditions – and the lack of dirt.

182

Without these bacterial challenges, it seems that a baby's immune system does not develop in a balanced way and, as a result, a whole generation becomes predisposed to allergies. Our understanding of what causes these long-term, chronic conditions is still really in its infancy and far more research is needed to uncover why it is that countries with different lifestyles see such different prevalence rates. Once we understand this, then we can look at factors such as diet or air pollution which may be exacerbating or causing the rates.

Genetic factors are also important and it's known that children with two parents who are both atopic are far more likely to develop an allergy as they grow up – although it may be an entirely different allergic condition. A huge amount of scientific research is involved in unravelling the different genetic factors. As this chapter was being written, scientists in Dundee, Scotland, announced that they had made yet another breakthrough on understanding the genetics behind eczema.

> Professor Irwin McLean and his team from the College of Medicine, Dentistry and Nursing at the University of Dundee, together with Dr Alan Irvine in Dublin, Ireland, have used a ground-breaking new method to examine the filaggrin gene. The team had reported in 2006 that defects in this particular gene can cause dry skin, eczema, eczema-associated asthma and other allergies.
>
> But their new work has shown that within the gene there can be several faults and that eczema sufferers of different ethnic backgrounds will have different faults within the gene.
>
> Their findings, published in *Nature* magazine, have found fifteen different mutations within the gene. One mutation in your gene means that you have a 60 per cent chance of having eczema. If you have two mutations in your gene, you have an almost 100 per cent chance of having eczema.

Of the mutations, five were prevalent in the European patients examined, who were mainly from the UK and Ireland, and 9 per cent of the population were shown to carry these gene defects. There are two mutations which are the most prevalent in all European people.

There were also two mutations prevalent in the Oriental populations that were tested. 4 per cent of people of Chinese descent carry this mutation, meaning it could lead to eczema in more than 50 million people in the Far East alone.

Eczema affects one in five children in the UK alone and is just as common in most parts of the world. The knowledge that Professor McLean's team is building will help them to develop a full picture of the disease, enable genetic testing and will take them a step closer to discovering new more effective treatments in years to come. Professor McLean said in a statement: 'Once we cracked this exceptionally difficult gene, we were surprised to learn how many different defects in filaggrin were waiting to be discovered, not only in European people, but other populations worldwide.'

In a clinic at the Royal Brompton Hospital in London, a number of adults are waiting for appointments with their specialist. Dr Andrew Menzies-Gow, a respiratory consultant specialising in asthma, is one of those who sees many patients who have tried and failed to keep their symptoms under control. He finds it alarming that so many of them spend years battling with the condition rather than getting proper help.

'There's something about asthma that means people just put up with it,' he explained. 'I don't understand why there is complacency. I suspect that because it doesn't generally kill people – although of course it can be fatal – it doesn't have a high profile. But asthma is affecting millions of people and we are not offering them a very good service.'

Asthma is a broad definition that covers many forms of the condition – some have an allergic trigger, and others do not. New therapies are being developed all the time. In March 2007, the news broke about a study of a completely new technique, known as bronchial thermoplasty, which volunteers said has made a huge improvement to their lives, enabling them to be more active.

The new treatment involves actually weakening the muscle around the airways and, in that way, reducing the contractions that cause pain and further damage. This weakening is achieved by inserting a fine tube into the airways and then heating their inner surface by using a heating element.

Professor Paul Corris, of Newcastle University, UK, said at the time: 'The treatment is not a replacement for drugs or inhalers, it is in conjunction with these other treatments. But the use of drugs and inhalers would be reduced as asthma attacks would become less common.'

184

Many doctors feel there is a need for better treatments that work more rapidly and are better tolerated. But currently, the mainstay of treatment is a range of medications which have to be taken in the right way, and that is also true for a number of other allergies. Patients tend to live with symptoms because they believe there are no better treatments available. That is not the case nowadays for hayfever, asthma or eczema, and despite the shortfalls in treatment, there are many thousands of people alive today who would not be here were it not for the newer treatments.

Educating yourself about your condition or your child's condition has to be your priority. Learning how to manage the condition is crucial to living with it. The key to all allergy control is self-management, and there are also many different patient groups to give you support and advice. Sometimes symptoms can change and you should never be scared to ask for help. As you'll have realised by now, there is a huge spectrum of medical opinion out there about allergies and sometimes it can seem hard to steer your way through it. Hopefully this book will have sorted out some of the facts from the fiction. Doctors are there to help, and whatever decisions you do come to about your condition, please ask their advice and work with them, as the biggest advances in treatment of allergies have come from mainstream medicine.

Many people will spend years not knowing exactly what causes their allergy and guess that it is cat fur, wool or house-dust mites, without ever going for a skin-prick test. In Britain, these should be available from every GP clinic, but they are not because too little money has gone into setting up the service. Many adult sufferers are under-treated and many never see a doctor or physician about their allergies. People tend to live with symptoms because they simply believe there are no better treatments available. I hope that this book will go some way towards making these conditions more easily understandable, and that it will be used to help people improve their quality of life by getting more accurate diagnoses and more effective treatment.

Glossary

Allergen A substance that is foreign to the body and can cause an allergic reaction in certain people. For example, pollen, dander.

Allergic contact dermatitis A red, itchy, weepy reaction where the skin has come into contact with a substance that provokes an immune reaction, such as nickel or latex.

Allergic rhinitis A medical term for hayfever. Symptoms include nasal congestion, a clear runny nose, sneezing, nose and eye itching and tearing eyes.

Allergy The immune system's misguided reaction to foreign substances, where it mistakes a harmless foreign body, such as a grain of pollen, for something dangerous.

Antibody A protein produced by the immune system to fight off particular invaders, known as antigens.

Anaphylaxis, or anaphylactic shock A severe allergic reaction which can be fatal if not treated properly.

Antigen A foreign body that creates an immune response.

Asthma A common allergy where chronic inflammation of the bronchial tubes in the lungs makes them swell, narrowing the airways. Symptoms can vary considerably, but include wheezing and breathlessness.

Atopic Being prone to allergies, or to do with an allergy.

Bacteria Single-celled organisms which can exist either as independent (free-living) organisms or as parasites (dependent upon another organism for life).

Basophil A white blood cell which is affected by the IgE antibody and plays a key role in allergic responses.

Bronchioles The small tubes within the lungs that enable us to breathe.

Bronchiolitis A viral infection of the lungs which affects babies and toddlers.

Bronchodilators A group of drugs that widen the airways in the lungs.

Bronchospasm The action of the muscles contracting suddenly around the airways.

Chronic A long-term medical condition.

Corticosteroids A group of anti-inflammatory drugs similar to the natural corticosteroid hormones produced in the body. They are used in the treatment of asthma.

Eczema A particular type of inflammatory reaction of the skin in which there is usually blisters on the skin at first, followed by erythema (reddening), edema (swelling), papules (bumps) and crusting of the skin. Usually begins in childhood and varies enormously in severity.

Histamine A substance that plays a major role in many allergic reactions. Histamine dilates blood vessels and makes the vessel walls abnormally permeable.

House-dust mite A tiny creature whose excretions cause an allergic reaction in many people. They live in most houses, in bedding and soft furnishings and are very hard to destroy.

Hypersensitivity An allergy, or allergic reaction, to something.

Immune Protected against infection.

Immune system The body's defence system, responsible for distinguishing us from everything foreign to us, and for protecting us against infections and foreign substances. When it goes awry, it starts to combat everyday substances such as pollen and particular foods.

Immunoglobulins Also known as antibodies, theses are proteins found in blood and in tissue fluids. Immunoglobulins are produced by cells of the immune system called B-lymphocytes.

Lymphocyte Any of a group of white blood cells of crucial importance to the adaptive part of the body's immune system. The adaptive portion of the immune system mounts a tailor-made defence when dangerous invading organisms penetrate the body's general defences.

Mast cell These play an important role in the body's allergic response. An allergen stimulates the release of antibodies, which attach themselves to mast cells.

Nebuliser A device that turns liquid therapy or drug into a fine mist which is then breathed in through a mask or mouthpiece.

RAST An abbreviation for RadioAllergoSorbent Test, a trademark of Pharmacia Diagnostics, which originated the test. RAST is a laboratory test used to detect IgE antibodies to specific allergens.

Respiratory system The group of organs responsible for carrying oxygen from the air to the bloodstream and for expelling the waste product carbon dioxide.

Rhinitis An inflammation of the nose.

Rhinorrhea The symptom of a runny nose.

Trachea The large airway, or tube, that leads down from the throat into the lungs.

Trigger A chemical or substance that sets off a disease in people who are genetically predisposed to developing the disease, or for someone with an allergy, that causes symptoms, e.g. birch pollen can be a trigger for hayfever sufferers.

Urticaria Another name for the hives. Raised, itchy areas of skin that are usually a sign of an allergic reaction.

Vaccines Therapies made of modified micro-organisms which stimulate an immune response in the body to prevent future infection with similar micro-organisms. They come in different forms, but are usually given by injection. Some last a lifetime, others have to be given every few years.

Venom Poison from an animal. For example, bee venom, snake venom, scorpion venom and spider venom.

Virus A micro-organism smaller than a bacteria, which cannot grow or reproduce apart from a living cell. A virus invades living cells and uses their chemical machinery to keep itself alive and to replicate itself.

Wheezing A whistling noise in the chest during breathing when the airways are narrowed or compressed.

Useful websites

Here are some reputable websites plus others which are interesting.

British Society for Allergy and Clinical Immunology
www.bsaci.org
This site lists all the NHS allergy clinics in Britain, as well as the doctors.

Allergy UK
www.allergyuk.org
The UK's leading charity for people with allergy, food intolerance and chemical sensitivity.

Asthma UK
www.asthma.org.uk
One of the biggest allergy organisations Part of the site is geared towards teenagers.

National Eczema Society
www.eczema.org
The main group in Britain helping patients and funding research into the condition.

www.rcplondon.ac.uk/pubs/brochure.aspx?e=11
The link for the excellent report on allergy services in the UK, written by the Royal College of Physicians.

National Institute of Allergy and Infectious Diseases
www3.niaid.nih.gov
Very good U.S. government website outlining the latest research.

edition.cnn.com/HEALTH/healthology
The excellent health library set up by CNN TV which contains video clips of experts talking about different allergies. Very digestible.

USEFUL WEBSITES

The Anaphylaxis Campaign
www.anaphylaxis.org.uk
The campaign group that was set up to give people more information about anaphylaxis, and which has contributed to improving warning systems on foods.

www.allergy-clinic.co.uk
A good website run by Dr Adrian Morris in Surrey, UK, who explains clearly what the various tests are for different allergies. Also gives a mainstream view of complementary therapies.

www.leapstudy.co.uk
The details for the major, seven-year study that is beginning at Guys' and St Thomas' Hospital, London, UK, to investigate the causes of peanut allergy.

ISAAC (the International Study of Asthma and Allergies in Childhood)
isaac.auckland.ac.nz
New Zealand based site for the worldwide research collaboration. Provides all the latest data on what is known in different countries.

The Global Allergy and Asthma European Network
www.ga2len.net
A consortium of leading European research centres specialising in allergic diseases. They have patient booklets to explain some of the conditions.

www.nhsdirect.nhs.uk
The British telephone and e-health information service which runs 24 hours a day. Gives clear information about symptoms and treatment and can put you in touch with doctors. Also available in several different languages.

www.bbc.co.uk/radio4/science/casenotes_20061024.shtml
One of BBC Radio 4's programmes investigating allergies. Dr Mark Porter reports on the conditions and looks at food allergies.

www.food.gov.uk/news/pressreleases/2007/mar/fsasmsalerts
Fantastic system that was launched as we were going to press. The Food Standards Agency has a new system which sends sufferers a text alert if a particular product is a risk to them.

environment.guardian.co.uk/food/story/0,,1828300,00.html
Link to a very good article by *Guardian* journalist Felicity Lawrence on how much soya there is in our diets.

Index